COPYRIGHT I

MW01594816

TABLE OF CONTENTS

INTRODUCTION

IS YOUR HEAD SPINNING WONDERING WHICH DIET TO TRY NEXT? BECAUSE IT DOESN'T SEEM LIKE ANY OF THEM WORK... TIRED OF DIETING ALL TOGETHER? DON'T WANT THE RESTRICT THEN BINGE CYCLE ANYMORE? SICK OF OVEREATING, BINGE EATING, OR EMOTIONAL EATING? TIRED OF FEELING OUT OF CONTROL AROUND FOOD? FEELING LIKE YOUR RELATIONSHIP WITH FOOD WILL NEVER CHANGE? JUST WANTING TO LOSE WEIGHT AND FEEL COMFORTABLE IN YOUR SKIN WITHOUT HAVING IT ALL BE SO DAMN HARD? I GET IT. I'VE BEEN THERE TOO! I WAS "GOOD" ALL DAY BUT CRAMMED MY FACE FULL OF COOKIES AND CHIPS IN THE PANTRY EVERY NIGHT. I WAS BLOATED, OVERWEIGHT, AND UNCOMFORTABLE IN MY BODY. I WAS FRUSTRATED, UNHAPPY, AND DIDN'T KNOW WHERE TO TURN TO CHANGE.

AS A KID I WAS NOT TAUGHT TO TUNE INTO MY BODY. I WASN'T TAUGHT TO LISTEN TO HUNGER AND FULLNESS OR TO TRUST MY BODY TO TELL ME WHAT IT NEEDS. I WAS TAUGHT TO OVERRIDE FULLNESS BY FINISHING MY PLATE. I LEARNED THAT FOOD WAS SCARCE SO YOU HAVE TO FINISH IT ALL. I LEARNED THAT EXERCISE WAS FOR LOSING WEIGHT AND IT WAS MADE TO BE TORTUROUS. IF YOU WEREN'T ACTIVELY TRYING TO MAKE YOUR BODY SMALLER THERE WAS NO POINT TO WORKING OUT.

I NOW KNOW THAT ALL THESE HABITS, BEHAVIORS, BELIEFS, AND PATTERNS ARE VERY INACCURATE. I WENT FROM WHERE YOU ARE NOW TO LOVING MY BODY, MOVING MY BODY IN WAYS THAT FEEL GOOD, LOSING WEIGHT AND MAINTAINING IT EFFORTLESSLY, BEING COMFORTABLE AROUND FOOD, NOT EATING MY EMOTIONS AND DEFINITELY NEVER STARTING OVER ON MONDAY (OR THE NEW YEAR) AGAIN! I WAS ABLE TO CHANGE MY RELATIONSHIP WITH FOOD, EXERCISE, AND BODY. BY CHANGING MY HABITS, BEING MINDFUL, AND TRUSTING MY BODY.

THIS BOOK IS THE GUIDE TO THAT FREEDOM. IT TEACHES YOU THE HABITS NECESSARY TO MAINTAIN A HEALTHY WEIGHT FOR YOU WITHOUT WEIGHING, MEASURING, OR COUNTING EVERYTHING THAT GOES INTO YOUR MOUTH. BECAUSE LET'S FACE IT... THAT IS NOT SOMETHING YOU WANT TO DO FOR THE REST OF YOUR LIFE! SO STOP DOING IT NOW! I WILL WALK YOU THROUGH THE STEPS I USED TO LOSE WEIGHT USING MINDFULNESS HABITS AND TUNING IN TO MY BODY'S CUES.

AS A HEALTH AND WELLNESS LIFE COACH, MY PASSION IS TO SEE AS MANY PEOPLE AS POSSIBLE CHANGE THEIR RELATIONSHIP WITH FOOD AND BODY FOR THE BETTER. I CREATED THIS JOURNAL SO THAT IN 16 WEEKS WITH CONSISTENT USE IT WILL HELP YOU LISTEN TO YOUR BODY, HEAL YOUR RELATIONSHIP WITH FOOD, AND BEST OF ALL, LOSE WEIGHT USING MINDFULNESS! IT IS YOUR PERSONAL TOOL FOR ACCOUNTABILITY AND MOTIVATION TO CREATE LASTING CHANGE.

WHAT EXACTLY IS MINDFULNESS?

MINDFULNESS IS USING ATTENTION AND AWARENESS TO BE IN THE PRESENT MOMENT. WE DO SO MANY THINGS OUT OF HABIT WITHOUT EVEN REGISTERING MENTALLY WHAT WE ARE DOING. WE JUST DO IT. THINGS LIKE SHOWERING, BRUSHING TEETH, DRIVING, AND EATING ARE ALL DONE WITH LITTLE THOUGHT TO THE ACTION WE ARE COMPLETING. BEING MINDFUL MEANS TO TURN OFF AUTOPILOT, GET OUT OF THE THOUGHTS AND EMOTIONS SWIRLING IN YOUR HEAD, AND BE FULLY IN THE NOW. IT'S FINDING CONTENTMENT AND PEACE AS YOU CHOOSE TO LET GO OF ANYTHING ELSE AND FOCUS ONLY ON THE TASK AT HAND. IT CAN BE UTILIZED IN ANY EVERYDAY TASK INCLUDING EATING, MOVEMENT, OR PLAYING WITH YOUR KIDS.

TO BE MINDFUL AT ANY POINT, WE HAVE TO FOCUS ON OUR FIVE SENSES. WE HAVE TO CONTEMPLATE WHAT WE FEEL, WHAT WE SEE, WHAT WE SMELL, TASTE, OR HEAR. WE HAVE TO NOTICE WE ARE WHIZZING THROUGH LIFE IN AUTOMATIC MODE AND CHOOSE TO BE PRESENT AND MINDFUL. CHOOSE TO LET GO OF THE TO DO LIST OR ANXIETY IN YOUR HEAD AND JUST BE HERE.

MINDFULNESS IS A MUSCLE TO FLEX. IT TAKES PRACTICE. MOST HUMANS CANNOT BE FULLY PRESENT OR MINDFUL AT EVERY MOMENT. BECAUSE LET'S FACE IT, THE PERK OF MEMORY IS THAT YOUR BRAIN INSTANTLY RECALLS HOW TO DO THINGS WITHOUT COMPREHENSION. AN EXAMPLE I LIKE TO USE IS DRIVING. WHEN WE FIRST LEARNED TO DRIVE WE HAD TO FOCUS ON EVERY DETAIL FROM PUTTING THE SEAT BELT ON TO SHIFTING THE CAR INTO DRIVE TO KNOWING WHEN TO ACCELERATE AND WHEN TO BRAKE. IN THIS EXAMPLE AND MANY OTHERS, WE NOW DO THINGS WITHOUT EVEN THINKING ABOUT THE EFFORT WE ARE PUTTING FORTH. BUT THIS AUTOMATICITY ALLOWS FOR OTHER THOUGHTS AND FEELINGS TO BE PRESENT THAT WE DON'T EVEN NECESSARILY NEED TO BE CONCERNED ABOUT AT THIS TIME. HAVE YOU EVER BEEN DEEP IN THOUGHT AND WONDERED WHY YOU ARE THINKING ABOUT THIS RIGHT NOW? THESE ARE THE MOMENTS THAT WE CAN CHOOSE TO BE MINDFUL AND ATTUNE TO WHAT'S GOING ON AROUND US.

DECIDING TO PRACTICE MINDFULNESS, ALLOWS YOU TO GET OUT OF YOUR HEAD AND INTO YOUR BODY. BEING IN YOUR BODY INSTEAD OF THE TORNADO OF THOUGHTS IN YOUR MIND LETS YOU EXPERIENCE THE MAGIC OF WHAT'S RIGHT IN FRONT OF YOU NOW. BECAUSE ULTIMATELY NOW IS ALL YOU HAVE. THE PAST IS A MEMORY AND THE FUTURE ISN'T HERE YET. IT'S ONLY NOW. THIS EXPERIENCE OF THE NOW MOMENT BRINGS PEACE AND CONTENTMENT FOR WHAT IS.

AGAIN A QUICK TOOL FOR INVOKING THIS SENSE OF SATISFACTION IMMEDIATELY IS BY NOTICING WHAT'S COMING IN THROUGH YOUR 5 SENSES. IT IS NEARLY IMPOSSIBLE TO BE IN YOUR HEAD'S SPIRALING THOUGHTS AND ALSO GIVING FULL CONSIDERATION TO WHAT IS GOING ON IN YOUR SURROUNDINGS. PAYING ATTENTION TO WHAT SOMETHING FEELS LIKE OR THE SMALL DETAILS OF IT'S LOOKS, OR THE TASTES/SMELLS, BRINGS YOU INTO THE NOW AND STOPS THE OVERACTIVE MIND CYCLE.

USING MINDFULNESS CAN HELP IN ANY AREA OF YOUR LIFE BUT THIS JOURNAL HELPS YOU USE IT SPECIFICALLY WITH EATING, MOVEMENT, YOUR BODY, AND NOTICING WHEN YOUR THOUGHTS ARE IN CHARGE. MINDFULNESS APPLIED TO THESE AREAS IS HOW YOU CREATE LASTING SHIFTS IN YOUR TIME ON THIS EARTH.

CHAPTER 1 GETTING STARTED

<u>HOW TO USE THIS BOOK</u>

IN THIS JOURNAL ONE CHAPTER EQUALS ONE HABIT. THE IDEA IS TO MASTER ONE HABIT AT A TIME SO AS TO NOT OVERWHELM. THIS ENSURES THE HABIT STICKS BEFORE MOVING ON TO THE NEXT.

CHAPTERS 4, 5, AND 6 ARE YOUR MAIN HABITS AND THEY REQUIRE THAT YOU WAIT IN BETWEEN READING THEM SO YOU CAN GET ONE DOWN BEFORE MOVING ON TO THE NEXT.

FOR CHAPTERS 4, 5, AND 6 ONLY YOU SHOULD READ AS THE BOOK PROMPTS. YOU WILL INCORPORATE ONE CHAPTER (ONE HABIT) AT A TIME, FILL OUT ALL THE JOURNAL PAGES FOR THAT HABIT AND WHEN THE ALLOTTED TIME OF HABIT INTEGRATION HAS PASSED, YOU WILL MOVE ON TO THE NEXT. IF ANY OF THIS SOUNDS CONFUSING, DON'T WORRY. AT THE END OF EACH CHAPTER YOU WILL BE GUIDED TO WHAT TO DO NEXT OR YOU CAN COME BACK TO THIS CHAPTER AND CHECK OFF WHERE YOU ARE AT.

▢ READ CHAPTERS 1, 2, 3, AND 4 TO START.
AFTER CHAPTER 4 THERE WILL BE PAGES FOR YOU TO BEGIN JOURNALING AND KEEPING TRACK OF HABITS. CHAPTER 4 IS FOCUSED ON EATING 3-4 MEALS A DAY WITH NO SNACKING IN BETWEEN. YOU WILL WORK ON THIS HABIT FOR 2 WEEKS BEFORE MOVING ON TO THE NEXT HABIT IN CHAPTER 5. AFTER 2 WEEKS WITH HABIT 1 IN CHAPTER 4 YOU WILL HAVE A GOOD GRASP ON EATING 3-4 MEALS PER DAY AND ARE READY TO MOVE ON.

▢ READ CHAPTER 5 AND INCORPORATE. SINCE CHAPTER 5 IS BASED ON RECOGNIZING HUNGER YOU WILL SPEND 3 TOTAL WEEKS ON THIS HABIT. ONE WEEK TO FOCUS ON HUNGER BEFORE EACH MEAL. ADD ON THE NEXT MEAL EACH WEEK.
▢ WEEK 1-ONE MEAL TO NOTICE HUNGER-RECOGNIZING HUNGER BEFORE BREAKFAST.
▢ WEEK 2-TWO MEALS NOTICING HUNGER- ADD IN RECOGNIZING HUNGER BEFORE LUNCH AND CONTINUE NOTICING HUNGER BEFORE BREAKFAST.
▢ WEEK 3-THREE MEALS NOTICING HUNGER- ADD IN RECOGNIZING HUNGER BEFORE DINNER AND CONTINUE NOTICING HUNGER BEFORE BREAKFAST AND LUNCH.

AFTER 3 WEEKS WITH CHAPTER 5, TIME TO MOVE ON TO THE NEXT HABIT.

█ READ CHAPTER 6 AND SPEND TWO WEEKS ON THE FULLNESS HABIT.

IMPORTANT TO NOTE-WHILE YOU'RE SPENDING WEEKS INCORPORATING HABITS, YOU MAY READ AHEAD TO CHAPTER 7 AND ANYTHING AFTER CHAPTER 7 INCLUDING APPENDIX A AND B WHERE YOU WILL FIND POSITIVE BODY IMAGE WORK AND RELAXATION TECHNIQUES. AGAIN FOLLOW THE PROMPTS AT THE END OF THE CHAPTERS TO KNOW WHAT THE COMING WEEKS WILL BRING.

OVERALL GOALS AND YOUR WHY

WE WILL START WITH WRITING DOWN YOUR OVERALL GOALS FOR BUYING THIS TRACKING JOURNAL AND YOUR WHY FOR GETTING THE WORK DONE.

- AS YOU WRITE YOUR GOALS THEY MUST INCLUDE THESE THINGS: ARE THEY SPECIFIC? LOSE WEIGHT IS NOT SPECIFIC ENOUGH. PICK A NUMBER SO IT CAN BE MEASURED HOW CLOSE YOU ARE TO YOUR GOAL. DO YOU ACTUALLY BELIEVE YOU CAN ACHIEVE IT? DON'T WRITE DOWN LOSE 100 POUNDS IF YOU DON'T BELIEVE IT'S POSSIBLE. STICK WITH SOMETHING THAT YOU DEEM REALISTIC. ONCE YOU'VE PROVEN TO YOURSELF WHAT IS POSSIBLE YOU CAN INCREASE THAT NUMBER LATER. THE FINAL STEP IS TO PUT A TIMELINE ON IT. PICK WHEN YOU WOULD LIKE TO ACHIEVE THIS GOAL BY. PUTTING TIME ON IT MEANS YOU HAVE TO GET TO DOING THE THINGS IN ORDER TO MAKE THAT GOAL HAPPEN IN THAT TIME FRAME. WITHOUT A GOAL DATE YOU WOULDN'T HAVE MOTIVATION AND YOU'D PUT IT OFF. SO YOUR GOALS NEED TO BE 1) SPECIFIC, 2) MEASURABLE, 3) BELIEVABLE, AND 4) TIMED.

NOW THAT YOU HAVE A SPECIFIC, MEASURABLE, BELIEVABLE GOAL AND YOU KNOW WHEN YOU WANT TO ACHIEVE THAT GOAL, WE WILL WORK ON YOUR WHY.

YOUR WHY IS YOUR MOTIVATION FOR DOING THIS. DO YOU WANT TO BE ABLE TO MOVE AROUND WITH YOUR KIDS WITHOUT GETTING WINDED? DO YOU WANT TO SEE YOUR GRANDKIDS GET MARRIED? DO YOU WANT TO FEEL COMFORTABLE IN YOUR BODY? DO YOU WANT TO SET A GOOD EXAMPLE FOR YOUR KIDS? THERE ARE A TON OF WHY'S OUT THERE. PICK YOURS AND BE SPECIFIC! "BEING HEALTHY" ISN'T SPECIFIC ENOUGH. WHY DO YOU WANT TO BE HEALTHY?

YOU WILL NOTICE THERE ARE WEEKLY OPPORTUNITIES TO WRITE YOUR WHY. THIS IS BECAUSE IT'S MOTIVATING. IT REMINDS YOU OF YOUR REASONS FOR MAKING THE CHOICE TO DO THE WORK AND STICK TO THE HABITS. SOMETIMES YOUR WHY CAN CHANGE. AS YOU GET TO WORK YOU MAY REALIZE SOME DEEPER REASONS AND YOU CAN CHANGE YOUR WHY LATER IN THE JOURNAL.

FILL IN YOUR CURRENT NUMBERS, GOALS AND YOUR WHY ON THE FOLLOWING PAGE. THEN READ CHAPTER 2.

FIRST THINGS FIRST...

DATE

MEASUREMENTS-   WEIGHT:

CHEST:

WAIST:

HIPS:

THIGHS: RIGHT-   LEFT-

CALF: RIGHT-   LEFT-

ARMS: RIGHT-   LEFT-

MY LONG TERM GOALS WHILE USING THIS JOURNAL: MAKE SURE IT'S SPECIFIC,
MEASURABLE, ACHIEVABLE, REALISTIC, AND TIMED.

_____

_____

_____

_____

_____

MY WHY AND MOTIVATION- WHY AM I TRYING TO REACH THESE GOALS?

_____

_____

_____

_____

_____

CHAPTER 2 MINDFUL EATING

MINDFUL EATING IS EATING WITH FOCUS AND ATTENTION. MINDFUL EATING INVOLVES TREATING A MEAL LIKE IT IS AN EXPERIENCE. YOU ARE HERE TO PARTICIPATE IN THIS ACTION OF EATING AND YOU WILL USE ALL YOUR SENSES TO DO IT. USING YOUR FIVE SENSES (SEE, HEAR, TASTE, TOUCH, AND SMELL) AT THE TABLE WHILE YOU EAT, MAKES YOU PRESENT IN THIS MOMENT. BEFORE EVEN TAKING A BITE YOU CAN BEGIN TO USE YOUR SENSES TO NOTICE AND QUESTION WHAT COLORS ARE ON MY PLATE? WHAT DOES IT SMELL LIKE? AS YOU DIG INTO THE FOOD YOU CAN GO OVER IN YOUR HEAD, WHAT DOES IT TASTE LIKE? WHAT FLAVORS DO I NOTICE? WHEN LOOKING FOR THINGS TO HEAR YOU CAN EITHER FOCUS ON THE SOUNDS AROUND YOU OR HOW IT SOUNDS DIFFERENT TO CHEW THE VARYING TEXTURES ON YOUR PLATE. FINALLY FOR FEELING OR TOUCH, WHAT TEXTURES ARE IN YOUR FOOD? IS IT SOFT, CRUNCHY, CHEWY, GRITTY, OR SMOOTH? TAKE NOTE OF ALL THESE THINGS AS YOU TUNE IN TO THE NOURISHMENT BEFORE YOU.

ANOTHER TOOL FOR FOCUSING ON YOUR MEAL IS TO THINK OF ITS ORIGIN AND ALL THE STEPS IT TOOK TO GET TO YOUR PLATE! TO ENGAGE IN THESE THOUGHTS IS ACTUALLY VERY MIND BLOWING! IF IT'S FRESH PRODUCE FOR EXAMPLE, IT HAS TO BE GROWN, HARVESTED, TAKEN TO THE PROCESSING PLANT, SHIPPED TO THE STORE AND BOUGHT BY YOU. THEN ANY PREPARATION YOU DID AT HOME! IF IT'S PACKAGED INSTEAD OF FRESH FOOD, THERE'S THE ADDED LAYER OF ALL THE STEPS THE FACTORY TAKES IN MAKING THE PRODUCT BEFORE SENDING IT TO THE STORE. WE REALLY ARE AN ABUNDANT SOCIETY AND ARE VERY LUCKY TO HAVE SO MUCH FOOD AND EASE AT OUR FINGERTIPS WHEN IT COMES TO MEALS! CAN YOU IMAGINE IF WE HAD TO GROW OR BUTCHER EVERYTHING WE ATE?? HAVING GRATITUDE FOR OUR ABILITY AND EASE TO HAVE FOOD IN OUR HOMES IS IMPORTANT TO CHANGING OUR RELATIONSHIP WITH FOOD.

Magnesium
Vitamin D
Omega-3

Prebiotic
w/ Pro and Postbiotic.
Collagen

OFTENTIMES AS WE SIT DOWN TO EAT A PLATE OF FOOD, WE ARE LOST IN THE HAPPENINGS OF THE DAY. OUR MINDS ARE A TORNADO OF THOUGHTS! HOW COULD SHE DO THIS?? THIS MORNING WAS TERRIBLE!! OR WE ARE DEEP IN SPECULATION REGARDING THE TO-DO LIST THAT STILL NEEDS TO BE DONE. DON'T FORGET TO LAY OUT THE MEAT FOR DINNER. OH WE HAVE BASEBALL TONIGHT! OR WE ARE PLAYING WITH OUR CELL PHONES AND WATCHING TV. THIS MAKES US NOT TUNE IN TO THE FOOD IN FRONT OF US. THIS LACK OF ATTENTIVENESS LEADS TO SWIFTLY FINISHING IT AND HAVING NO RECOLLECTION OF IT EVEN GOING INTO OUR MOUTH. DANG! DID I EVEN EAT?? THIS IS WHERE OVEREATING COMES IN BECAUSE WE WILL HEAD BACK FOR SECONDS OR THE PANTRY FOR A SNACK SINCE THE MEAL WASN'T VERY SATISFYING. BUT OUR BODIES DON'T NEED MORE FOOD, IT'S JUST THAT OUR BRAIN WAS SO BUSY, WE DIDN'T REGISTER THE CONSUMPTION OF FOOD AND THE FULLNESS IT PROVIDED.

MINDFUL EATING BRINGS AWARENESS TO THE MEAL SO YOU DON'T OVEREAT. AFTER A BUSY MORNING OR FATIGUING DAY, IT CAN BE CHALLENGING TO BRING YOURSELF INTO AWARENESS BEFORE YOU BEGIN TO TAKE BITES. BUT I'VE GOT YOU COVERED, HEAD OVER TO APPENDIX B FOR BREATHING AND FOCUSING TECHNIQUES THAT CAN HELP YOU CALM YOUR MIND IN ORDER TO BE ABLE TO ENJOY THE FOOD IN FRONT OF YOU. ALL THE TECHNIQUES IN APPENDIX B WILL PROVIDE A SENSE OF FOCUSING ON THE HERE AND NOW SO YOU CAN BE PRESENT WITH YOUR FOOD AND ENJOY WITHOUT OVERDOING IT. THE OVERCONSUMPTION IS WHAT GETS YOU AWAY FROM YOUR WEIGHT LOSS GOALS. AND MOST IMPORTANTLY ALWAYS TURN OFF THE TV AND LEAVE YOUR PHONE SOMEWHERE ELSE WHILE YOU EAT AT THE TABLE TO AVOID THE DISTRACTION OF ELECTRONICS.

SOMETIMES EATING TOO FAST GETS IN THE WAY OF EATING MINDFULLY SO IN ORDER TO SLOW YOURSELF DOWN I RECOMMEND PUTTING THE FORK DOWN IN BETWEEN BITES. IF YOU ARE QUICK TO PICK IT BACK UP, TRY COUNTING TO TEN IN BETWEEN BITES. SO ONCE YOU FINISH CHEWING A BITE, COUNT TO TEN BEFORE PICKING UP YOUR FORK TO TAKE ANOTHER, AND YOU'LL SET YOUR FORK DOWN AFTER THE BITE ONCE AGAIN.

CHAPTER 3 MINDSET

YOUR MINDSET IS A KEY PLAYER IN WHETHER YOUR GOALS WILL BE ACHIEVED OR NOT. YOUR BRAIN IS LIKE A COMPUTER. WE INSTALL THE PROGRAMS. SO INSTALL ONES THAT ARE GOOD AND BENEFICIAL TO WEIGHT LOSS. WE CHANGE THE PROGRAMMING AND BELIEFS BY SETTING GOALS, USING AFFIRMATIONS, AND VISUALIZATIONS. ALL THINGS THAT THIS JOURNAL HAS IN IT. THE NEW PROGRAM YOU'RE WORKING ON INSTALLING INTO YOUR BRAIN LEADS TO NEW BELIEFS. NEW BELIEFS LEAD TO NEW ACTIONS. NEW ACTIONS RESULT IN THE BODY CHANGE YOU DESIRE. CHANGING THE INSIDE LANDSCAPING, THOUGHTS AND BELIEFS, IS JUST AS IMPORTANT AS CHANGING THE OUTSIDE. THE INSIDE HAS TO BE CHANGED FIRST. YOU HAVE TO CONVINCE YOURSELF THAT THIS CAN ACTUALLY HAPPEN IN ORDER FOR IT TO.

LIMITING BELIEFS ARE CONSISTENT THOUGHTS WE THINK THAT ACTUALLY HOLD US BACK FROM REACHING A GOAL. WE HAVE SO MANY LIMITING BELIEFS AROUND WEIGHT LOSS AND BODY TRANSFORMATION BECAUSE WE'VE TRIED OTHER DIETS AND PROGRAMS THAT WERE UNSUCCESSFUL. THESE ATTEMPTS JUST BURNED THESE BELIEFS EVEN DEEPER INTO OUR HARD DRIVE. OUR LIMITING BELIEFS ARE THE THINGS WE TELL OURSELVES FREQUENTLY LIKE WEIGHT LOSS IS HARD, MY METABOLISM IS TOO SLOW, I HAVE BAD GENES, I JUST CAN'T EXERCISE LIKE OTHER PEOPLE, I DON'T HAVE TIME, I HAVE NO CONTROL AROUND FOOD AND SO MANY OTHERS THAT DON'T SERVE US. BUT I LIKE TO THINK OF THOSE PAST EXPERIENCES AS LEARNING OPPORTUNITIES RATHER THAN FAILURES. THEY HAVE TAUGHT YOU WHAT DOESN'T WORK. SO THANK THEM FOR THAT EXPERIENCE AND LET THEM GO. WE ARE MOVING INTO A NEW WAY OF THINKING AND BEING THAT WILL MOVE THE NEEDLE TOWARD THE WAY YOU WANT TO BE.

IN THE NEXT FEW PAGES THERE WILL BE TWO JOURNAL PAGES TO FILL OUT TO GET TO THE ROOT OF YOUR BELIEFS AND REFRAME THEM TO BE POSITIVE AFFIRMATIONS. WE WILL BE SWITCHING FROM THE NEGATIVE MINDSET OF "I CAN'T DO THIS BECAUSE ..." TO POSITIVE EMPOWERING THOUGHTS THAT ARE MOTIVATING. MAKING THIS CHANGE IN BELIEFS IS THE FIRST STEP IN GETTING UNSTUCK FROM YOUR CURRENT PATTERNS AND HABITS AROUND BODY TRANSFORMATION. AS YOU CHANGE THE WAY YOU THINK, YOU BEGIN TO TAKE ACTION AND SHOW UP IN NEW WAYS AS WELL. THE ACTION PORTION IS WHERE THE MAGIC HAPPENS. YOU BEGIN TO BE THE PERSON THAT VALUES THEIR BODY, CHOOSES TO MOVE IT BECAUSE IT FEELS GOOD, AND NOURISHES IT WITH FOOD THAT SERVES.

BELIEFS ARE ONLY TRUE BECAUSE YOU KEEP THINKING THEM. CHANGE YOUR BELIEFS TO CHANGE YOUR BODY!

OTHER JOURNAL PAGES FOLLOWING THIS CHAPTER INCLUDE "NEW ME VS OLD ME" AND "IT'S ALREADY HERE!" THESE PAGES SERVE TO MOTIVATE YOU AND GET YOU EXCITED TO GET TO WORK. REPEAT THESE JOURNAL PROMPTS FREQUENTLY AND ADD THEM TO THIS BOOK TO LOOK BACK ON LATER!

PRO-TIP: TAKE TIME TO CURATE YOUR SOCIAL MEDIA FEED TO BE UPLIFTING, MOTIVATING, AND ENCOURAGING. FOLLOW PEOPLE THAT DO THOSE EXACT THINGS TO BUILD YOU UP WHILE YOU SCROLL. UNFOLLOW THE PEOPLE THAT ONLY MAKE YOU GET CAUGHT IN A COMPARISON TRAP AND THEREFORE UNHAPPY. YOU CAN FIND ME AT SHELBY A ADKINS ON ALL THE SOCIALS IF YOU ARE LOOKING FOR SOME POSITIVE PEOPLE.

DO THE FOLLOWING JOURNAL PAGES THEN READ CHAPTER 4.

BELIEFS

WRITE DOWN YOUR BELIEFS ABOUT HOW WEIGHT LOSS AND BODY CHANGE WORKS
FOR YOU? WHY DOESN'T IT WORK? IS IT EASY OR HARD? DO YOU FAIL AND START
OVER A LOT? WHAT OTHER REASONS DO YOU HAVE FOR NOT REACHING THE GOALS
YOU SET? DIG INTO WHAT YOU BELIEVE IS HOLDING YOU BACK AND LIST IT ALL BELOW.
WRITE DOWN EVERY EXCUSE THAT COMES TO MIND.

_____

_____

_____

_____

_____

_____

_____

_____

_____

_____

_____

_____

_____

_____

_____

ON THE NEXT PAGE, YOU WILL REWRITE THESE THOUGHTS TO BE POSITIVE AND
PRODUCTIVE. THIS WILL BEGIN TO REPROGRAM THE BELIEF SYSTEM IN YOUR BRAIN.
THE REPROGRAMMING WILL EMPOWER YOU TO START TAKING ACTION IN ORDER TO
MEET YOUR GOALS.

AFFIRMATIONS

USING YOUR BELIEFS FROM THE PREVIOUS PAGE, CREATE POSITIVE AND PRODUCTIVE STATEMENTS (AKA AFFIRMATIONS). TURN THOSE NEGATIVE THOUGHTS INTO POWERFUL PHRASES TO CHANGE YOUR MINDSET AROUND BODY TRANSFORMATION.

_____

EX: I AM MAKING CHOICES TO HAVE VIBRANT HEALTH
_____

EX: I LOSE WEIGHT WITH EASE, I AM TAKING STEPS THAT LEAD TO SUCCESS
_____

EX: I TRUST MY BODY AND I HAVE THE POWER TO CHANGE MY EATING HABITS
_____

EX: I AM PUTTING IN THE WORK TO MEET MY GOALS
_____

EX: I AM WORTHY OF WEIGHT LOSS
_____

_____

_____

_____

_____

_____

_____

_____

_____

_____

_____

_____

YOU WILL PICK ONE OR TWO TO WRITE ON YOUR DAILY JOURNAL PAGE. IF YOU DON'T HAVE ENOUGH ROOM TO WRITE THEM ALL DAILY, STICK WITH THE SAME ONE OR TWO FOR AT LEAST 2 WEEKS BEFORE CHANGING TO ANOTHER. WE WANT TO MAKE SURE ONE BELIEF STICKS BEFORE ADDING MORE.

NAMING THE PLAYERS

THIS JOURNAL PAGE WILL BRING AWARENESS TO THE CHARACTERS IN YOUR HEAD THAT EFFECT THE WAY YOU FEEL AND INTERACT WITH FOOD AND YOUR BODY. DIG DEEP, THINK OF ALL THE NEGATIVE PEOPLE AND LIST THEM BELOW WITH THEIR ROLE.

EX: DEB THE DIETER-ALWAYS SAYING "DON'T EAT THAT, YOU'LL GAIN WEIGHT"

EX: BODY IMAGE BETTY- BODY CHECKS IN THE MIRROR, MAKES NEGATIVE COMMENTS

EX: IMPULSIVE IRMA- INSISTS ON EATING BEYOND FULLNESS, "JUST ONE MORE BITE"

EX: THE GIVE UPPER, THE ALL OR NOTHING'ER, THE BINGE/EMOTIONAL EATER

THE GOAL OF THIS ACTIVITY IS TO GET YOU TO NOTICE WHEN THOSE THOUGHTS IN YOUR HEAD ARE EFFECTING YOUR RELATIONSHIP WITH FOOD AND BODY. IN RECOGNIZING THESE "VOICES" YOU CAN BEGIN TO DISAGREE WITH THEM.
EX: "NO DEB I CAN TRUST MY BODY TO USE THE FOOD I TAKE IN AND NOT GAIN WEIGHT
NO BETTY- MY BODY IS AMAZING, IT DOES SO MUCH!!
NO IRMA-WE CAN HAVE MORE LATER, WE DO NOT NEED TO OVEREAT.

OLD ME VS NEW ME

IN THIS JOURNAL SESSION YOU WILL LIST THE WAYS YOU'VE CHANGED IN YOUR LIFE, WITH FOOD AND BODY, CAREER, RELATIONSHIPS, ANYTHING! IT CAN BE DONE TWO WAYS: 1) IT CAN BE WRITTEN IN CURRENT TIME. MEANING "OLD ME" IS HOW YOU ARE NOW AND "NEW ME" IS HOW YOU WILL BE ONCE YOU REACH YOUR GOALS OR 2) ONCE YOU HAVE MADE SOME POSITIVE CHANGES IN ANY AREA OF YOUR LIFE YOU CAN WRITE IT LOOKING BACK TO SEE HOW FAR YOU'VE COME! "OLD ME" IS HOW YOU USED TO BE AND "NEW ME" IS HOW YOU ARE NOW. BOTH WAYS ARE GREAT AND SERVE TO MOTIVATE! DOING THESE PROMPTS MORE THAN ONCE IS VERY HELPFUL, FEEL FREE TO WRITE THEM ON A BLANK PIECE OF PAPER.

OLD ME:

_____

_____

_____

_____

_____

_____

_____

NEW ME:

_____

_____

_____

_____

_____

_____

IT'S ALREADY HERE!!

IN THIS JOURNAL SESSION, YOU WILL WRITE DOWN WHAT IT WILL BE LIKE WHEN YOU HAVE REACHED YOUR FOOD AND BODY GOALS. BE SPECIFIC! WHAT WILL YOU BE WEARNG? HOW WILL YOU FEEL PHYSICALLY AND MENTALLY? ARE YOU MORE COMFORTABLE SHOWING UP IN PLACES YOU HAVEN'T BEFORE? HOW ARE YOU IN RELATIONSHIPS OR AT WORK? DO THIS PROMPT OFTEN TO REALLY FEEL HOW IT WILL BE! THIS FEELING WILL EMPOWER YOU TO KEEP GOING TOWARDS YOUR GOAL.

_____

_____

_____

_____

_____

_____

_____

_____

_____

_____

_____

_____

_____

_____

_____

_____

_____

_____

RELATIONSHIP WITH THE SCALE

I THINK I SPEAK FOR MOST IN SAYING THAT OUR RELATIONSHIP WITH THE SCALE CAN BE LESS THAN FAVORABLE. IT TENDS TO BE SOMETHING THAT CAN AFFECT OUR WHOLE DAY. IF IT SHOWS WHAT WE WANT, THEN THE DAY IS GOOD. WE ARE GOOD. IF IT ISN'T EXACTLY WHAT WE'D PREFER, THE DAY IS BAD, OUR EFFORTS HAVE BEEN FOR NOTHING AND WE BASICALLY SUCK.

LET'S PUT THE SCALE IN ITS PLACE... IT'S A SQUARE THAT MEASURES GRAVITY PUSHING AGAINST IT FOR GOODNESS SAKE. THE SCALE SHOULD NOT BE AFFECTING YOU NEGATIVELY. THERE ARE SO MANY THINGS THAT CAN SKEW THE NUMBER LIKE MENSTRUATION, BOWEL MOVEMENTS, SALT AND WATER INTAKE, OR MEDICATION. IT'S JUST ONE TOOL TO SHOW YOUR PROGRESS. MORE IMPORTANTLY THAN THAT NUMBER IS HOW YOU FEEL MENTALLY AND PHYSICALLY OR HOW YOUR CLOTHES ARE FITTING.

SO YES, THIS IS A BOOK AND JOURNAL TO PROMOTE WEIGHT LOSS BUT THAT DOESN'T MEAN THAT A NUMBER BETWEEN YOUR FEET COMING FROM A BOX ON THE FLOOR HAS ANY REFLECTION OF YOUR SELF-WORTH. YOU ARE WORTHY AND AMAZING JUST AS YOU ARE. NOTICE YOUR THOUGHTS AND REACTIONS TO THE NUMBER WHEN YOU WEIGH IN. IF THEY ARE NEGATIVE THOUGHTS, HOW CAN YOU REFRAME THEM? RECOGNIZE WHEN A THOUGHT IS GOING TO HELP OR HURT YOUR DAY. TURN TO YOUR AFFIRMATIONS AND STATE TO YOURSELF THAT YOU ARE CHANGING! THE BODY ACHIEVES WHAT THE MIND BELIEVES. DON'T LET THE SCALE MAKE YOU BELIEVE ANYTHING NEGATIVE ABOUT YOURSELF.

ALSO KEEP IN MIND THAT WEIGHT LOSS IS NOT GOING TO BE STRAIGHT DOWN. IT WILL ALWAYS FLUCTUATE. AND A FEW POUNDS ONE WAY OR THE OTHER DOESN'T MEAN YOU ARE OR ARE NOT DOING GOOD WORK TO NORMALIZE YOUR RELATIONSHIP WITH FOOD. DON'T MAKE THE NUMBER MEAN SOMETHING PERSONALLY ABOUT YOU. YOU ARE WHOLE, COMPLETE, AND LOVEABLE JUST AS YOU ARE.

I HOPE YOU GET TO A POINT IN YOUR JOURNEY THAT YOU TRUST YOUR BODY ENOUGH TO STOP THE CONSISTENT WEIGHING IN. JUST KNOW THAT BY STICKING TO THE HABITS AND DOING THE WORK, YOU ARE CREATING TRANSFORMATION.

CHAPTER 4 HABIT 1
EATING 3-4 MEALS PER DAY, NO SNACKING

THIS HABIT IS THE BEGINNING OF YOUR NEW WAY OF BEING WITH FOOD. IT REALLY HELPS YOU NOTICE WHEN YOU EAT MINDLESSLY OR SNACK RELATED TO HABIT RATHER THAN OUT OF HUNGER. IT WAKES YOU UP TO GRABBING CANDY BARS FROM THE DISH AT WORK MULTIPLE TIMES A DAY OR MUNCHING ON COOKIES OR A BAG OF CHIPS DURING THAT AFTERNOON SLUMP. EATING CAN HAPPEN WITHOUT THOUGHT BUT THIS HABIT BRINGS IT BACK AROUND TO EATING 3-4 MODERATELY SIZED MEALS DURING THE DAY WHICH SERVES OUR BODY AND WEIGHT LOSS GOALS.

NO MORE SMALL MEALS 6 TIMES A DAY OR GRABBING FOOD WITHOUT THINKING. NO MORE CARRYING AROUND GRANOLA BARS AND TRAIL MIX JUST IN CASE YOU GET HUNGRY. WE ARE GOING FOR 3-4 WELL ROUNDED MEALS THAT HAVE PROTEIN, CARB, AND FAT. THIS BOOK WON'T GO HEAVY INTO NUTRITION BUT HAVING ALL THE MAIN COMPONENTS KEEPS YOU FULLER LONGER SO YOU CAN MAKE IT 3-4 HOURS IN BETWEEN MEALS WHICH RESULTS IN ONLY EATING 3-4 TIMES A DAY INSTEAD OF FREQUENT CONSUMPTION. HAVING AN UNBALANCED MEAL MEANS YOU WILL BE HUNGRIER SOONER. FOOD IS THE FUEL THAT KEEPS YOU GOING AND YOUR BODY DESERVES TO EAT.

THESE MEALS WILL BE PLATED AND ENJOYED DISTRACTION FREE LIKE MENTIONED IN THE MINDFUL EATING CHAPTER. ANYTHING THAT YOU PLAN TO CONSUME SHOULD BE ON YOUR PLATE, EVEN DESSERT, SO YOU ARE AWARE OF WHAT YOU ARE CONSUMING. TAKING TASTES, EATING FROM A KIDS PLATE, AND NIBBLING WHILE YOU PICK UP AFTER DINNER ARE ALL HABITS THAT MOVE US FURTHER FROM WEIGHT LOSS. SO PLATE EVERYTHING. DO NOT TAKE A BITE UNLESS IT'S ON YOUR PLATE!

TIMING YOUR MEALS-MOSTLY YOUR MEALS SHOULD BE SPACED 3-4 HOURS APART. IF YOU EAT BREAKFAST AND ARE HUNGRY 2 HOURS LATER, LOOK BACK AT YOUR BREAKFAST. DID IT HAVE ALL THE FOOD GROUPS? DID YOU EAT ENOUGH? SOMETIMES WE ARE USED TO EATING SMALL MEALS AND THEY JUST DON'T LAST LONG. JUST KNOW THAT THIS IS PRACTICE AND TAKES TIME. EACH MEAL THAT YOU INVESTIGATE WHY YOU GOT HUNGRY SOONER THAN USUAL, BRINGS YOU CLOSER TO KNOWING WHAT YOUR BODY NEEDS TO LOSE WEIGHT, WITHOUT BEING HUNGRY ALL THE TIME.

ANOTHER AREA TO CLARIFY IS THE NEED FOR A FOURTH MEAL VERSUS JUST THREE. SOMETIMES WE GET UP SUPER EARLY WHICH MEANS AN EARLY BREAKFAST, AN EARLY LUNCH, AND THEN DINNER SEEMS LIKE A LONG WAY AWAY. THAT IS WHEN I'D THROW IN AN AFTERNOON "MEAL" SO I AM NOT RAVENOUS BY TIME DINNER ROLLS AROUND. IF YOU ARE OVERLY HUNGRY BY THE TIME DINNER OR ANY MEAL FOR THAT MATTER ROLLS AROUND, YOU ARE MORE LIKELY TO ENGAGE IN EATING BEHAVIORS THAT GET US FARTHER FROM OUR GOALS. FOR EXAMPLE EATING FROM THE PANTRY OR EATING FOOD WITHOUT PLATING IT TENDS TO HAPPEN WHEN WE ARE TOO HUNGRY. ALL OF THESE HABITS KEEP US FROM REACHING OUR GOALS BECAUSE WE AREN'T AWARE OF HOW MUCH WE ARE CONSUMING. SO IF YOU HAVE DAYS THAT REQUIRE A FOURTH MEAL, HAVE A LATE AFTERNOON ONE. AGAIN THIS WILL BE BALANCED WITH PROTEIN, CARB AND FAT BECAUSE THIS IS A MEAL NOT A SNACK. THIS FOURTH MEAL IS THE ONLY INSTANCE THAT YOU COULD HAVE IT BE SMALLER IN ORDER TO BE HUNGRY FOR DINNER. WE WILL GET TO HUNGER AND FULLNESS IN LATER CHAPTERS SO DON'T WORRY ABOUT IT TOO MUCH FOR NOW, JUST FOCUS ON 3-4 MEALS A DAY AND NOTHING IN BETWEEN.

WHEN IT COMES TO ALCOHOL AND HIGH CALORIE COFFEES OR DRINKS, THESE CAN BE CONSIDERED SNACKS BECAUSE OF THEIR CALORIE DENSENESS. IF YOU CONSUME THEM IN MODERATION, ENJOY THEM WITH MEALS SO YOU CAN STILL REACH YOUR GOALS. IF THEY ARE ENJOYED OUTSIDE OF MEALS, THEY WILL SKEW HUNGER AND FULLNESS CUES WHICH WILL COME IN THE NEXT HABITS AND CHAPTERS.

NOW GET TO WORK MAKING THE HABIT OF EATING 3-4 MEALS PER DAY YOUR NORM! SINCE YOU WILL BE WORKING ON THIS HABIT FOR 2 WEEKS, THERE WILL BE 14 JOURNAL PAGES (ONE DAILY) FOR THIS HABIT. YOU WILL COMPLETE ALL 14 BEFORE MOVING ON TO THE NEXT CHAPTER'S HABIT. THERE IS ALSO A WEEKLY JOURNAL SHEET THAT COMES IN AFTER 7 DAYS OF HABIT WORK. THE WEEKLY SHEET HAS DIFFERENT PROMPTS AFTER YOU HAVE COMPLETED THE WEEK AND KEEPS YOU MOTIVATED SO MAKE SURE TO BE FILLING IN ALL THIS GOOD INFO!

DURING THE 2 WEEKS OF WORKING ON THIS HABIT AND DOING THE PROVIDED DAILY JOURNAL SHEET, YOU CAN GO TO CHAPTER 7 OR ANY CHAPTER AFTER THAT FOR CONTINUED READING. YOU MAY ALSO GO TO APPENDIX A OR B TO WORK ON POSITIVE BODY IMAGE PRACTICES AND RELAXATION TECHNIQUES. CHAPTERS 4, 5, AND 6 BUILD ON EACH OTHER SO FOR BEST RESULTS IT IS RECOMMENDED TO NOT MOVE ON TO CHAPTER 5 OR 6 UNTIL YOU HAVE COMPLETED THE FULL TWO WEEKS OF HABIT 1.

REMEMBER THIS IS A MARATHON, NOT A SPRINT. THIS IS HOW YOU CHANGE YOUR RELATIONSHIP WITH FOOD FOREVER!

HAPPY HABITING!

HOW TO USE THE DAILY JOURNAL PAGE

THE DAILY JOURNAL PAGE IS YOUR PARTNER IN STAYING MOTIVATED! IT HAS EVERYTHING YOU NEED TO TRACK AND WRITE DOWN. REMEMBER TO RECORD EVERYTHING! YOU'LL BE ABLE TO LOOK BACK ON THIS AND SEE A PATTERN OF EATING, SLEEPING, WATER, MOVEMENT, ETC AND HOW IT ALL TIES TOGETHER.

1)TO DO LIST: ANYTHING YOU NEED A REMINDER TO COMPLETE TODAY

2)TODAY I AM GRATEFUL FOR: LIST 2 OR MORE THINGS THAT YOU ARE GRATEFUL FOR TODAY. SOMETHING AS SEEMINGLY SMALL AS A WARM CUP OF COFFEE OR AS BIG AS SOMEONE HELPING YOU CHANGE A FLAT TIRE.

3)DAILY AFFIRMATION: YOUR POSITIVE STATEMENT FOR REPROGRAMMING YOUR BRAIN FROM THE PREVIOUS JOURNAL PAGES.

4)CRAVINGS AND REACTIONS: THIS IS WHEN YOU REALLY WANT FOOD AND YOU AREN'T HUNGRY. WRITE DOWN WHAT YOU WANTED AND HOW YOU HANDLED IT. EVEN IF YOU DIDN'T NAVIGATE IT THE WAY YOU WOULD PREFER, WRITE IT DOWN SO YOU CAN DO BETTER NEXT TIME. MAYBE YOU TRIED SOMETHING BUT IT DIDN'T WORK. WRITE IT ALL DOWN TO LOOK BACK ON LATER.

5)WATER TRACKER: AIM FOR AT LEAST 8 GLASSES OF WATER A DAY AND CHECK THEM OFF AS YOU GO!

6)MOVEMENT: WRITE DOWN HOW YOU MOVED YOUR BODY TODAY. WALK, YOGA, GYM, WEIGHTS, SWIMMING. WRITE SOMETHING DOWN HERE EVERY DAY! WE ARE MADE TO MOVE!

DAILY JOURNAL

DATE

TO DO LIST:

_____

_____

_____

TODAY I AM GRATEFUL FOR:

1.

_____

2.

_____

DAILY AFFIRMATION:

_____

CRAVINGS AND MY REACTION TO THEM

_____

_____

_____

_____

WATER TRACKER ◊◊◊◊◊◊◊

MOVEMENT

_____

MOOD TRACKER ☹ ☹ ☺ ☺ ☺

HOURS OF SLEEP:

3-4 MEALS, NO SNACKING YES/NO

_____

_____

_____

DAILY FOOD OR BODY WIN

_____

_____

_____

INTENTION SETTING FOR TOMORROW

_____

_____

_____

DAILY JOURNAL

DATE

TO DO LIST:

_____

_____

_____

TODAY I AM GRATEFUL FOR:

1. _____

2. _____

DAILY AFFIRMATION:

_____

CRAVINGS AND MY REACTION TO THEM

_____

_____

_____

_____

INTENTION SETTING FOR TOMORROW

_____

_____

_____

WATER TRACKER ⬠⬠⬠⬠⬠⬠⬠

MOVEMENT

_____

MOOD TRACKER ☹ ☹ 😐 ☺ 😊

HOURS OF SLEEP:

3-4 MEALS, NO SNACKING   YES/NO

_____

_____

_____

DAILY FOOD OR BODY WIN

_____

_____

_____

_____

DAILY JOURNAL

DATE

TO DO LIST:

WATER TRACKER 　◇◇◇◇◇◇◇

MOVEMENT

MOOD TRACKER 　😣 😟 😐 😊 😊

TODAY I AM GRATEFUL FOR:

HOURS OF SLEEP:

1.

3-4 MEALS, NO SNACKING 　　　YES/NO

2.

DAILY AFFIRMATION:

CRAVINGS AND MY REACTION TO THEM

DAILY FOOD OR BODY WIN

INTENTION SETTING FOR TOMORROW

DAILY JOURNAL

DATE

TO DO LIST:

WATER TRACKER ◇◇◇◇◇◇◇

MOVEMENT

MOOD TRACKER ☹ ☹ 😐 ☺ ☺

TODAY I AM GRATEFUL FOR:

HOURS OF SLEEP:

1.

3-4 MEALS, NO SNACKING   YES/NO

2.

DAILY AFFIRMATION:

CRAVINGS AND MY REACTION TO THEM

DAILY FOOD OR BODY WIN

INTENTION SETTING FOR TOMORROW

DAILY JOURNAL

DATE

TO DO LIST:

WATER TRACKER ◇◇◇◇◇◇◇

MOVEMENT

MOOD TRACKER 😫 😟 😐 🙂 😊

TODAY I AM GRATEFUL FOR:

HOURS OF SLEEP:

1.

3-4 MEALS, NO SNACKING YES/NO

2.

DAILY AFFIRMATION:

CRAVINGS AND MY REACTION TO THEM

DAILY FOOD OR BODY WIN

INTENTION SETTING FOR TOMORROW

DAILY JOURNAL

DATE

TO DO LIST:

_____

_____

_____

TODAY I AM GRATEFUL FOR:

1. _____

2. _____

DAILY AFFIRMATION:

_____

CRAVINGS AND MY REACTION TO THEM

_____

_____

_____

_____

WATER TRACKER ⬡⬡⬡⬡⬡⬡⬡

MOVEMENT

_____

_____

MOOD TRACKER ☹ ☹ 😐 ☺ ☺

HOURS OF SLEEP:

3-4 MEALS, NO SNACKING   YES/NO

_____

_____

_____

DAILY FOOD OR BODY WIN

_____

_____

_____

_____

INTENTION SETTING FOR TOMORROW

_____

_____

_____

_____

WEEKLY JOURNAL

DATE

WEIGHT:

MY WHY...

_____

_____

_____

_____

WHAT IS GOING WELL WITH THIS WEEKS HABIT?

_____

_____

_____

WHAT COULD BE BETTER?

_____

_____

_____

GOALS FOR NEXT WEEK...

_____

_____

_____

DAILY JOURNAL

DATE

TO DO LIST:

_____

_____

_____

TODAY I AM GRATEFUL FOR:

1.

_____

2.

_____

DAILY AFFIRMATION:

_____

CRAVINGS AND MY REACTION TO THEM

_____

_____

_____

_____

WATER TRACKER ⬭⬭⬭⬭⬭⬭⬭

MOVEMENT

_____

MOOD TRACKER ☹ ☹ 😐 ☺ 😊

HOURS OF SLEEP:

3-4 MEALS, NO SNACKING   YES/NO

_____

_____

_____

DAILY FOOD OR BODY WIN

_____

_____

_____

_____

INTENTION SETTING FOR TOMORROW

_____

_____

_____

DAILY JOURNAL

DATE

TO DO LIST:

_____

_____

_____

TODAY I AM GRATEFUL FOR:

1. _____

2. _____

DAILY AFFIRMATION:

_____

CRAVINGS AND MY REACTION TO THEM

_____

_____

_____

WATER TRACKER   ◇◇◇◇◇◇◇

MOVEMENT

_____

MOOD TRACKER   ☹ ☹ ☺ ☺ ☺

HOURS OF SLEEP:

3-4 MEALS, NO SNACKING   YES/NO

_____

_____

_____

DAILY FOOD OR BODY WIN

_____

_____

_____

INTENTION SETTING FOR TOMORROW

_____

_____

DAILY JOURNAL

DATE

TO DO LIST:

WATER TRACKER ◊◊◊◊◊◊◊

MOVEMENT

MOOD TRACKER 😣 😟 😐 🙂 😊

TODAY I AM GRATEFUL FOR:

HOURS OF SLEEP:

1.

3-4 MEALS, NO SNACKING   YES/NO

2.

DAILY AFFIRMATION:

CRAVINGS AND MY REACTION TO THEM

DAILY FOOD OR BODY WIN

INTENTION SETTING FOR TOMORROW

DAILY JOURNAL

DATE

TO DO LIST:

WATER TRACKER ◊◊◊◊◊◊◊

MOVEMENT

MOOD TRACKER ☹ ☹ ☺ ☺ ☺

TODAY I AM GRATEFUL FOR:

HOURS OF SLEEP:

1.

3-4 MEALS, NO SNACKING   YES/NO

2.

DAILY AFFIRMATION:

CRAVINGS AND MY REACTION TO THEM

DAILY FOOD OR BODY WIN

INTENTION SETTING FOR TOMORROW

DAILY JOURNAL

DATE

TO DO LIST:

WATER TRACKER ⬡⬡⬡⬡⬡⬡⬡

MOVEMENT

TODAY I AM GRATEFUL FOR:

MOOD TRACKER ☹ ☹ ☺ ☺ ☺

HOURS OF SLEEP:

1.

3-4 MEALS, NO SNACKING   YES/NO

2.

DAILY AFFIRMATION:

CRAVINGS AND MY REACTION TO THEM

DAILY FOOD OR BODY WIN

INTENTION SETTING FOR TOMORROW

DAILY JOURNAL

DATE _____

TO DO LIST:
_____

_____

_____

_____

TODAY I AM GRATEFUL FOR:

1. _____

_____

2. _____

_____

DAILY AFFIRMATION:
_____

CRAVINGS AND MY REACTION TO THEM
_____

_____

_____

_____

_____

WATER TRACKER ⬦⬦⬦⬦⬦⬦⬦

MOVEMENT
_____

_____

MOOD TRACKER ☹ ☹ ☺ ☺ ☺

HOURS OF SLEEP:

3-4 MEALS, NO SNACKING   YES/NO

_____

_____

_____

_____

DAILY FOOD OR BODY WIN
_____

_____

_____

_____

INTENTION SETTING FOR TOMORROW
_____

_____

_____

DAILY JOURNAL

DATE

TO DO LIST:

WATER TRACKER ⬦⬦⬦⬦⬦⬦⬦

MOVEMENT

MOOD TRACKER ☹ ☹ 😐 ☺ 😊

TODAY I AM GRATEFUL FOR:

HOURS OF SLEEP:

1.

3-4 MEALS, NO SNACKING   YES/NO

2.

DAILY AFFIRMATION:

CRAVINGS AND MY REACTION TO THEM

DAILY FOOD OR BODY WIN

INTENTION SETTING FOR TOMORROW

WEEKLY JOURNAL

DATE

WEIGHT:

MY WHY...

_____
_____
_____
_____

WHAT IS GOING WELL WITH THIS WEEKS HABIT?

_____
_____
_____
_____

WHAT COULD BE BETTER?

_____
_____
_____
_____

GOALS FOR NEXT WEEK...

_____
_____
_____
_____

CHAPTER 5 HABIT 2
RECOGNIZING HUNGER

THE ULTIMATE GOAL OF THIS HABIT IS TO GET YOU TO 1) NOTICE HUNGER, 2) KNOW WHEN IT IS REAL HUNGER INSTEAD OF HEAD HUNGER AND 3) WAIT 30-60 MINUTES FROM THE TIME OF NOTICING THAT HUNGER TO WHEN YOU ACTUALLY SIT DOWN TO CONSUME FOOD. WAITING WITH HUNGER FOR 30-60 MINUTES BEFORE EATING IS WHERE THE MAGIC HAPPENS. OVER TIME THIS WAITING PERIOD CREATES THE ENERGY DEFICIT NEEDED FOR WEIGHT LOSS. INSTANT CONSUMPTION WHEN HUNGRY MEANS YOU EAT MORE FREQUENTLY AND DO NOT MEET GOALS.

HUNGER IS OUR FRIEND. IT IS THE BODY'S WAY OF TELLING US IT'S TIME TO INTAKE MORE FOOD. THROUGH HUNGER THE BODY SAYS I'VE USED ALL THE PREVIOUSLY INGESTED NUTRIENTS AND I NEED MORE TO FUEL OUR EXISTENCE. IN OUR YEARS OF DIETING WE HAVE TENDED TO OVERRIDE THIS BASIC PHYSIOLOGICAL SENSATION IN ORDER TO MEET OUR WEIGHT LOSS GOALS. CHOOSING TO TUNE BACK INTO HUNGER AND MAKE IT OUR ALLY IS HOW WE CAN LOSE OR MAINTAIN WEIGHT WITHOUT USING BRAIN POWER TO COUNT CALORIES, CARBS, OR MACROS. YOUR BODY IS A CALORIE COUNTER IN ITSELF AND HUNGER IS REASSURANCE THAT YOU HAVE USED UP THE LAST MEAL AND IT'S TIME FOR MORE!

FOR THOSE OF US THAT HAVE SPENT DECADES IGNORING, HATING, AND NOT TRUSTING HUNGER, TUNING IN TO THIS SENSATION CAN BE CHALLENGING. THERE ARE DIFFERENCES TO NOTE BETWEEN PHYSICAL HUNGER AND MENTAL HUNGER. DIFFERENTIATING REAL HUNGER FROM FAKE HUNGER IS A PRACTICE BUT HERE'S SOME WAYS TO LEARN TO TELL THEM APART.

TRUE HUNGER COMES ON GRADUALLY AND IT HAS A PHYSICAL FEELING IN YOUR BODY. THE EASIEST WAY TO DESCRIBE HOW TRUE HUNGER FEELS IS AN EMPTY SENSATION IN YOUR UPPER ABDOMEN. IT CAN BE FOLLOWED BY THE HUNGRY GURGLING OF IT IF YOU HAVE WAITED LONG ENOUGH BETWEEN MEALS.

WHEN WORKING ON MASTERING THE HABIT OF RECOGNIZING HUNGER, YOU'LL BEGIN TO NOTICE THE FEELING OF HUNGER, THEN THINK TO YOURSELF "OK, I SEEM TO BE GETTING A LITTLE HUNGRY". AFTER CONSIDERING THIS AS POTENTIALLY REAL HUNGER THEN START TO INVESTIGATE TO DETERMINE ITS VALIDITY. QUESTIONS YOU CAN ASK YOURSELF INCLUDE: "WHEN DID I LAST EAT?" "WAS IT BALANCED AND DECENT SIZED OR DID I HAVE ONLY ONE FOOD GROUP?"

DEPENDING ON HOW LONG AGO YOU ATE, SAY IT WAS ONLY ONE HOUR AGO, MAY PROVE IF YOU'RE PHYSICALLY HUNGRY OR MENTALLY HUNGRY. IF YOU ATE 1 HOUR AGO, YOU SHOULD NOT BE HUNGRY AGAIN JUST YET. ONCE YOU'VE FIGURED OUT WHEN YOUR LAST MEAL WAS, YOU'LL WAIT OUT THE HUNGER. REAL HUNGER WILL GET STRONGER IN THE NEXT 15-30 MINUTES. IF IT DOESN'T GET STRONGER THEN IT WASN'T TRUE HUNGER.

ANYTIME WE GET THE FEELING OF HUNGER WE WAIT 30-60 MINUTES TO MAKE SURE IT'S REAL. IN THIS TIME OF WAIT, BEGIN TO PLAN WHAT BALANCED MEAL YOU WILL HAVE AND DRINK A GLASS OF WATER. THIS PAUSE TO CHECK FOR REAL HUNGER GIVES YOU THE OPPORTUNITY TO PLAN SOMETHING THAT NOURISHES RATHER THAN QUICK GRABBING FOR FOOD THAT DOESN'T SERVE YOUR BODY AND LEAVES YOU DESIRING MORE. PLUS THE EXTRA HYDRATION WILL LET YOU KNOW IF YOUR BODY WAS JUST NEEDING WATER AND NOT FOOD. IF IT DOESN'T GET STRONGER YOU DON'T HAVE TO EAT AND YOU HAVE GIVEN YOURSELF SOME PRACTICE AT RECOGNIZING TRUE HUNGER. GOOD WORK!

SOMETIMES WE MAY THINK WE ARE HUNGRY BUT IT ISN'T OUR BODY THAT IS IN NEED OF FOOD. THIS IS HEAD HUNGER. HEAD HUNGER IS A TYPE OF EMOTIONAL EATING. YOU ARE NOT PHYSICALLY HUNGRY BUT FOOD WOULD PROVIDE SOME COMFORT AT THIS POINT AND YOU ARE DESIRING IT. SOMETIMES FOOD GIVES YOU AN EXCUSE TO STOP WORKING OR IF YOU'RE UPSET BY SOMETHING THAT CAN MAKE YOU WANT FOOD FOR COMFORT. A STRONG WAY TO TELL THE DIFFERENCE BETWEEN REAL HUNGER AND HEAD HUNGER IS WHAT YOU ARE HUNGRY FOR. HEAD HUNGER WANTS A SPECIFIC FOOD. SOMETHING FROM THE PANTRY, SOMETHING PACKAGED, ESPECIALLY THE SALTY OR SWEET VARIETIES.

A GOOD TEST TO TELL WHETHER IT'S REAL HUNGER OR HEAD HUNGER IS TO ASK YOURSELF IF YOU WOULD EAT AN APPLE OR SOME BROCCOLI RIGHT NOW. CHANCES ARE THAT IF YOU WOULD EAT A BALANCED HEALTHY MEAL AT THIS MOMENT YOU ARE ACTUALLY PHYSICALLY HUNGRY. IF YOU ARE ONLY HUNGRY FOR COOKIES AND CHIPS, THAT'S MOST LIKELY A HEAD HUNGER OR EMOTIONAL DESIRE TO EAT AND WE WILL DIVE MORE INTO THAT IN A DIFFERENT CHAPTER. FOR NOW, I AM TRYING TO GET YOU TO NOTICE THE DIFFERENCE BETWEEN REAL PHYSICAL HUNGER AND HEAD HUNGER/EMOTIONAL EATING. THE GOAL IS TO NOT EAT UNLESS IT'S ACTUAL PHYSICAL HUNGER. THIS HABIT OF RECOGNIZING AND EATING ONLY WHEN HUNGRY ALLOWS YOU TO SEE WHEN YOU USE FOOD FOR EMOTIONS AND BOREDOM.

IMPORTANT THING TO NOTE ABOUT HUNGER... IT IS NOT AN EMERGENCY! I KNOW A LOT OF PEOPLE ARE LIKE "OH NO, I'M GETTING HUNGRY, I MUST HAVE FOOD NOW!" HUNGER IS A GOOD THING! IT'S A PHYSICAL REMINDER OF A NEED.

FOR EXAMPLE WHEN YOU GET TIRED IN THE EVENING, THERE'S NOTHING WRONG WITH IT, IT JUST MEANS YOU WILL GO TO BED SOON. SAME WAY WITH HUNGER. IT JUST MEANS YOU NEED TO BEGIN THINKING OF YOUR NEXT MEAL. IT'S JUST AN INNER PROMPTING SYSTEM. LISTENING TO THIS PROMPTING SYSTEM IS WHERE WEIGHT LOSS GETS EASIER! LETTING YOUR BODY LEAD THE WAY SUPPORTS A HEALTHY WEIGHT WITHOUT RESTRICTING. WE KNOW WHEN WE RESTRICT, WE WILL TEND TO EXPERIENCE THE DOWNSIDES OF THAT RESTRICTION LATER, LIKE BINGE EATING, OVEREATING AND GUILT.

YOU WILL BE WORKING ON RECOGNIZING HUNGER AND WAITING 30-60 MINUTES BEFORE EATING FOR A TOTAL OF 3 WEEKS. EACH WEEK WILL FOCUS ON NOTICING HUNGER BEFORE A SPECIFIC MEAL AND ADD ON ANOTHER MEAL THE FOLLOWING WEEK. WEEK ONE IS FOR NOTICING HUNGER BEFORE BREAKFAST. WEEK TWO YOU WILL ADD LUNCH HUNGER TO THE BREAKFAST HUNGER YOU HAVE ALREADY MASTERED. WEEK THREE YOU WILL ADD DINNER HUNGER TO THE OTHER TWO MEALS YOU'VE BEEN WORKING ON. IF YOU'RE HAVING A FOURTH MEAL, MAKE SURE YOU ARE UTILIZING THIS HABIT HERE AS WELL.

SINCE THIS HABIT IS 3 WEEKS LONG, THERE WILL BE 21 JOURNAL PAGES (ONE DAILY) FOR THIS HABIT. YOU WILL COMPLETE ALL 21 BEFORE MOVING ON TO THE NEXT CHAPTER'S HABIT. THERE IS ALSO A WEEKLY JOURNAL SHEET THAT COMES IN AFTER 7 DAYS OF HABIT WORK.

A MONTHLY JOURNAL SHEET WILL ALSO COME IN DURING THIS 3 WEEK HABIT SINCE IT WILL HAVE BEEN 4 WEEKS SINCE YOU HAVE STARTED YOUR MINDFUL EATING JOURNEY. THIS MONTHLY JOURNAL PAGE ALLOWS YOU TO WRITE DOWN SOME MEASUREMENTS OF YOUR BODY AND REFLECT BACK ON HOW FAR YOU'VE COME! GIVE YOURSELF A PAT ON THE BACK! HABIT CHANGE CREATES LASTING DEVELOPMENT AND YOU'VE GOT THIS!!

DAILY JOURNAL

DATE

TO DO LIST:

_____

_____

_____

WATER TRACKER ⬦⬦⬦⬦⬦⬦⬦

MOVEMENT

_____

_____

MOOD TRACKER ☹ ☹ ☺ ☺ ☺

TODAY I AM GRATEFUL FOR:

1.

_____

2.

_____

HOURS OF SLEEP:

3-4 MEALS, NO SNACKING   YES/NO

HUNGER 30 MINUTES BEFORE BREAKFAST   YES/NO

_____

_____

DAILY AFFIRMATION:

_____

CRAVINGS AND MY REACTION TO THEM

_____

_____

_____

_____

DAILY FOOD OR BODY WIN

_____

_____

_____

_____

INTENTION SETTING FOR TOMORROW

_____

_____

_____

DAILY JOURNAL

DATE

TO DO LIST:

_____

_____

_____

TODAY I AM GRATEFUL FOR:

1. _____

_____

2. _____

_____

DAILY AFFIRMATION:

_____

CRAVINGS AND MY REACTION TO THEM

_____

_____

_____

_____

WATER TRACKER   ○○○○○○○

MOVEMENT

_____

MOOD TRACKER   ☹ ☹ ☺ ☺ ☺

HOURS OF SLEEP:

3-4 MEALS, NO SNACKING   YES/NO

HUNGER 30 MINUTES BEFORE BREAKFAST   YES/NO

_____

_____

_____

DAILY FOOD OR BODY WIN

_____

_____

_____

INTENTION SETTING FOR TOMORROW

_____

_____

_____

DAILY JOURNAL

DATE

TO DO LIST:

_____

_____

_____

_____

TODAY I AM GRATEFUL FOR:

1. _____

_____

2. _____

_____

DAILY AFFIRMATION:

_____

CRAVINGS AND MY REACTION TO THEM

_____

_____

_____

_____

WATER TRACKER ◊◊◊◊◊◊◊

MOVEMENT

_____

MOOD TRACKER ☹ ☹ ☺ ☺ ☺

HOURS OF SLEEP:

3-4 MEALS, NO SNACKING	YES/NO

HUNGER 30 MINUTES BEFORE BREAKFAST	YES/NO

_____

_____

_____

DAILY FOOD OR BODY WIN

_____

_____

_____

_____

INTENTION SETTING FOR TOMORROW

_____

_____

_____

_____

DAILY JOURNAL

DATE

TO DO LIST:

WATER TRACKER ◇◇◇◇◇◇◇

MOVEMENT

MOOD TRACKER ☹ ☹ 😐 🙂 😊

TODAY I AM GRATEFUL FOR:

HOURS OF SLEEP:

1.

3-4 MEALS, NO SNACKING   YES/NO

2.

HUNGER 30 MINUTES BEFORE BREAKFAST   YES/NO

DAILY AFFIRMATION:

CRAVINGS AND MY REACTION TO THEM

DAILY FOOD OR BODY WIN

INTENTION SETTING FOR TOMORROW

DAILY JOURNAL

DATE

TO DO LIST:

WATER TRACKER ⬡⬡⬡⬡⬡⬡⬡

MOVEMENT

MOOD TRACKER ☹ ☹ ☺ ☺ ☺

TODAY I AM GRATEFUL FOR:

HOURS OF SLEEP:

1.

3-4 MEALS, NO SNACKING   YES/NO

HUNGER 30 MINUTES BEFORE BREAKFAST   YES/NO

2.

DAILY AFFIRMATION:

CRAVINGS AND MY REACTION TO THEM

DAILY FOOD OR BODY WIN

INTENTION SETTING FOR TOMORROW

DAILY JOURNAL

DATE

TO DO LIST:

WATER TRACKER ⬦⬦⬦⬦⬦⬦⬦

MOVEMENT

MOOD TRACKER ☹ ☹ ☺ ☺ ☺

TODAY I AM GRATEFUL FOR:

HOURS OF SLEEP:

1.

3-4 MEALS, NO SNACKING   YES/NO

HUNGER 30 MINUTES BEFORE BREAKFAST   YES/NO

2.

DAILY AFFIRMATION:

CRAVINGS AND MY REACTION TO THEM

DAILY FOOD OR BODY WIN

INTENTION SETTING FOR TOMORROW

DAILY JOURNAL

DATE

TO DO LIST:

_____

_____

_____

_____

TODAY I AM GRATEFUL FOR:

1. _____

_____

2. _____

_____

DAILY AFFIRMATION:

_____

_____

CRAVINGS AND MY REACTION TO THEM

_____

_____

_____

_____

_____

WATER TRACKER ◇◇◇◇◇◇◇◇

MOVEMENT

_____

_____

MOOD TRACKER ☹ ☹ ☺ ☺ ☺

HOURS OF SLEEP:

3-4 MEALS, NO SNACKING   YES/NO

HUNGER 30 MINUTES BEFORE BREAKFAST   YES/NO

_____

_____

_____

_____

DAILY FOOD OR BODY WIN

_____

_____

_____

_____

INTENTION SETTING FOR TOMORROW

_____

_____

_____

WEEKLY JOURNAL

WEIGHT:

MY WHY...

_____

_____

_____

_____

WHAT IS GOING WELL WITH THIS WEEKS HABIT?

_____

_____

_____

WHAT COULD BE BETTER?

_____

_____

_____

GOALS FOR NEXT WEEK...

_____

_____

_____

DAILY JOURNAL

DATE

TO DO LIST:

_____

_____

_____

TODAY I AM GRATEFUL FOR:

1. _____

_____

2. _____

_____

DAILY AFFIRMATION:

_____

CRAVINGS AND MY REACTION TO THEM

_____

_____

_____

_____

WATER TRACKER   ○○○○○○○

MOVEMENT

_____

MOOD TRACKER   ☹ ☹ ☺ ☺ ☺

HOURS OF SLEEP:

3-4 MEALS, NO SNACKING	YES/NO
HUNGER 30 MINUTES BEFORE BREAKFAST	YES/NO
HUNGER 30 MIN BEFORE LUNCH	YES/NO

_____

_____

DAILY FOOD OR BODY WIN

_____

_____

_____

_____

INTENTION SETTING FOR TOMORROW

_____

_____

_____

DAILY JOURNAL

DATE

TO DO LIST:

_____

_____

_____

TODAY I AM GRATEFUL FOR:

1. _____

2. _____

DAILY AFFIRMATION:

_____

CRAVINGS AND MY REACTION TO THEM

_____

_____

_____

_____

WATER TRACKER   ◊◊◊◊◊◊◊◊

MOVEMENT

_____

MOOD TRACKER   ☹ ☹ ☺ ☺ ☺

HOURS OF SLEEP:

3-4 MEALS, NO SNACKING   YES/NO

HUNGER 30 MINUTES BEFORE BREAKFAST   YES/NO

HUNGER 30 MIN BEFORE LUNCH   YES/NO

_____

_____

DAILY FOOD OR BODY WIN

_____

_____

_____

INTENTION SETTING FOR TOMORROW

_____

_____

_____

DAILY JOURNAL

DATE

TO DO LIST:

_____

_____

_____

_____

TODAY I AM GRATEFUL FOR:

1. _____

_____

2. _____

_____

DAILY AFFIRMATION:

_____

CRAVINGS AND MY REACTION TO THEM

_____

_____

_____

_____

INTENTION SETTING FOR TOMORROW

_____

_____

_____

WATER TRACKER ◇◇◇◇◇◇◇

MOVEMENT

_____

_____

MOOD TRACKER ☹ ☹ ☺ ☺ ☺

HOURS OF SLEEP:

3-4 MEALS, NO SNACKING   YES/NO

HUNGER 30 MINUTES BEFORE BREAKFAST   YES/NO

HUNGER 30 MIN BEFORE LUNCH   YES/NO

_____

_____

DAILY FOOD OR BODY WIN

_____

_____

_____

_____

DAILY JOURNAL

DATE

TO DO LIST:

_____

_____

_____

TODAY I AM GRATEFUL FOR:

1. _____

_____

2. _____

_____

DAILY AFFIRMATION:

_____

CRAVINGS AND MY REACTION TO THEM

_____

_____

_____

_____

INTENTION SETTING FOR TOMORROW

_____

_____

_____

WATER TRACKER ◊◊◊◊◊◊◊

MOVEMENT

_____

MOOD TRACKER ☹ ☹ ☺ ☺ ☺

HOURS OF SLEEP:

3-4 MEALS, NO SNACKING   YES/NO

HUNGER 30 MINUTES BEFORE BREAKFAST   YES/NO

HUNGER 30 MIN BEFORE LUNCH   YES/NO

_____

_____

DAILY FOOD OR BODY WIN

_____

_____

_____

DAILY JOURNAL

DATE

TO DO LIST:

WATER TRACKER   ⬭⬭⬭⬭⬭⬭⬭

MOVEMENT

MOOD TRACKER   ☹ ☹ ☺ ☺ ☺

TODAY I AM GRATEFUL FOR:

HOURS OF SLEEP:

1.

3-4 MEALS, NO SNACKING   YES/NO

HUNGER 30 MINUTES BEFORE BREAKFAST   YES/NO

2.

HUNGER 30 MIN BEFORE LUNCH   YES/NO

DAILY AFFIRMATION:

CRAVINGS AND MY REACTION TO THEM

DAILY FOOD OR BODY WIN

INTENTION SETTING FOR TOMORROW

DAILY JOURNAL

DATE

TO DO LIST:

_____

_____

_____

TODAY I AM GRATEFUL FOR:

1. _____

2. _____

_____

DAILY AFFIRMATION:

_____

CRAVINGS AND MY REACTION TO THEM

_____

_____

_____

_____

WATER TRACKER   ○○○○○○○

MOVEMENT

_____

MOOD TRACKER   ☹ ☹ ☺ ☺ ☺

HOURS OF SLEEP:

3-4 MEALS, NO SNACKING   YES/NO

HUNGER 30 MINUTES BEFORE BREAKFAST   YES/NO

HUNGER 30 MIN BEFORE LUNCH   YES/NO

_____

_____

DAILY FOOD OR BODY WIN

_____

_____

_____

_____

INTENTION SETTING FOR TOMORROW

_____

_____

_____

DAILY JOURNAL

DATE

TO DO LIST:

WATER TRACKER   ○○○○○○○

MOVEMENT

MOOD TRACKER   ☹ ☹ ☺ ☺ ☺

TODAY I AM GRATEFUL FOR:

HOURS OF SLEEP:

1.

3-4 MEALS, NO SNACKING   YES/NO

HUNGER 30 MINUTES BEFORE BREAKFAST   YES/NO

2.

HUNGER 30 MIN BEFORE LUNCH   YES/NO

DAILY AFFIRMATION:

CRAVINGS AND MY REACTION TO THEM

DAILY FOOD OR BODY WIN

INTENTION SETTING FOR TOMORROW

WEEKLY JOURNAL

WEIGHT:

MY WHY...

_____

_____

_____

_____

WHAT IS GOING WELL WITH THIS WEEKS HABIT?

_____

_____

_____

_____

WHAT COULD BE BETTER?

_____

_____

_____

_____

GOALS FOR NEXT WEEK...

_____

_____

_____

_____

MONTHLY JOURNAL

DATE

MEASUREMENTS-

CHEST:

WAIST:

HIPS:

THIGHS: RIGHT-   LEFT-

CALF: RIGHT-   LEFT-

ARMS: RIGHT-   LEFT-

LOOK HOW FAR I'VE COME!!
WRITE DOWN EXAMPLES OF WAYS YOU HAVE IMPROVED IN THE LAST 4 WEEKS

_____

_____

_____

_____

_____

_____

_____

_____

_____

_____

DAILY JOURNAL

DATE

TO DO LIST:

_____

_____

_____

TODAY I AM GRATEFUL FOR:

1. _____

2. _____

DAILY AFFIRMATION:

_____

CRAVINGS AND MY REACTION TO THEM

_____

_____

_____

_____

INTENTION SETTING FOR TOMORROW

_____

_____

_____

WATER TRACKER ◊◊◊◊◊◊◊

MOVEMENT

_____

MOOD TRACKER ☹ ☹ 😐 ☺ ☺

HOURS OF SLEEP:

3-4 MEALS, NO SNACKING   YES/NO

HUNGER 30 MINUTES BEFORE BREAKFAST   YES/NO

HUNGER 30 MIN BEFORE LUNCH   YES/NO

HUNGER 30 MIN BEFORE DINNER   YES/NO

DAILY FOOD OR BODY WIN

_____

_____

_____

_____

DAILY JOURNAL

DATE

TO DO LIST:

WATER TRACKER ○○○○○○○

MOVEMENT

TODAY I AM GRATEFUL FOR:

MOOD TRACKER ☹ ☹ ☺ ☺ ☺

HOURS OF SLEEP:

1.

3-4 MEALS, NO SNACKING   YES/NO

HUNGER 30 MINUTES BEFORE BREAKFAST   YES/NO

2.

HUNGER 30 MIN BEFORE LUNCH   YES/NO

HUNGER 30 MIN BEFORE DINNER   YES/NO

DAILY AFFIRMATION:

CRAVINGS AND MY REACTION TO THEM

DAILY FOOD OR BODY WIN

INTENTION SETTING FOR TOMORROW

DAILY JOURNAL

DATE

TO DO LIST:

_____

_____

_____

TODAY I AM GRATEFUL FOR:

1. _____

_____

2. _____

_____

DAILY AFFIRMATION:

_____

CRAVINGS AND MY REACTION TO THEM

_____

_____

_____

_____

WATER TRACKER ⬡⬡⬡⬡⬡⬡⬡

MOVEMENT

_____

MOOD TRACKER ☹ 🙁 😐 🙂 😊

HOURS OF SLEEP:

3-4 MEALS, NO SNACKING	YES/NO
HUNGER 30 MINUTES BEFORE BREAKFAST	YES/NO
HUNGER 30 MIN BEFORE LUNCH	YES/NO
HUNGER 30 MIN BEFORE DINNER	YES/NO

_____

DAILY FOOD OR BODY WIN

_____

_____

_____

_____

INTENTION SETTING FOR TOMORROW

_____

_____

_____

DAILY JOURNAL

DATE

TO DO LIST:

WATER TRACKER ⬡⬡⬡⬡⬡⬡⬡

MOVEMENT

MOOD TRACKER ☹ ☹ 😐 🙂 😊

TODAY I AM GRATEFUL FOR:

HOURS OF SLEEP:

1.

3-4 MEALS, NO SNACKING   YES/NO

HUNGER 30 MINUTES BEFORE BREAKFAST   YES/NO

2.

HUNGER 30 MIN BEFORE LUNCH   YES/NO

HUNGER 30 MIN BEFORE DINNER   YES/NO

DAILY AFFIRMATION:

CRAVINGS AND MY REACTION TO THEM

DAILY FOOD OR BODY WIN

INTENTION SETTING FOR TOMORROW

DAILY JOURNAL

DATE

TO DO LIST:

WATER TRACKER ◊◊◊◊◊◊◊

MOVEMENT

MOOD TRACKER ☹ ☹ ☺ ☺ ☺

TODAY I AM GRATEFUL FOR:

HOURS OF SLEEP:

1.

3-4 MEALS, NO SNACKING   YES/NO

HUNGER 30 MINUTES BEFORE BREAKFAST   YES/NO

2.

HUNGER 30 MIN BEFORE LUNCH   YES/NO

HUNGER 30 MIN BEFORE DINNER   YES/NO

DAILY AFFIRMATION:

CRAVINGS AND MY REACTION TO THEM

DAILY FOOD OR BODY WIN

INTENTION SETTING FOR TOMORROW

DAILY JOURNAL

DATE

TO DO LIST:

_____

_____

_____

_____

TODAY I AM GRATEFUL FOR:

1. _____

_____

2. _____

_____

DAILY AFFIRMATION:

_____

CRAVINGS AND MY REACTION TO THEM

_____

_____

_____

_____

WATER TRACKER ⬡⬡⬡⬡⬡⬡⬡

MOVEMENT

_____

_____

MOOD TRACKER ☹ ☹ 😐 ☺ ☺

HOURS OF SLEEP:

3-4 MEALS, NO SNACKING   YES/NO

HUNGER 30 MINUTES BEFORE BREAKFAST   YES/NO

HUNGER 30 MIN BEFORE LUNCH   YES/NO

HUNGER 30 MIN BEFORE DINNER   YES/NO

_____

DAILY FOOD OR BODY WIN

_____

_____

_____

_____

INTENTION SETTING FOR TOMORROW

_____

_____

_____

DAILY JOURNAL

DATE

TO DO LIST:

WATER TRACKER   ⬡⬡⬡⬡⬡⬡⬡

MOVEMENT

MOOD TRACKER   ☹ 🙁 😐 🙂 😊

TODAY I AM GRATEFUL FOR:

HOURS OF SLEEP:

3-4 MEALS, NO SNACKING	YES/NO

1.

HUNGER 30 MINUTES BEFORE BREAKFAST	YES/NO

HUNGER 30 MIN BEFORE LUNCH	YES/NO

2.

HUNGER 30 MIN BEFORE DINNER	YES/NO

DAILY AFFIRMATION:

CRAVINGS AND MY REACTION TO THEM

DAILY FOOD OR BODY WIN

INTENTION SETTING FOR TOMORROW

WEEKLY JOURNAL

DATE

WEIGHT:

MY WHY...
_____
_____
_____
_____

WHAT IS GOING WELL WITH THIS WEEKS HABIT?
_____
_____
_____
_____

WHAT COULD BE BETTER?
_____
_____
_____
_____

GOALS FOR NEXT WEEK...
_____
_____
_____
_____

CHAPTER 6 HABIT 3
NOTICING FULLNESS

THE HABITS FROM THE LAST FEW WEEKS AND NOW THIS CHAPTER IS ABOUT TUNING IN TO YOUR BODY, LISTENING, AND ALLOWING IT TO GUIDE YOU. WHEN WE TUNE IN, IT GETS EASIER! WE DON'T EAT ACCORDING TO A CLOCK OR BY COUNTING OUT WHAT WE THINK OUR BODY NEEDS. WE NATURALLY EAT WHEN WE ARE HUNGRY AND STOP WHEN WE HAVE HAD JUST ENOUGH.

OUR FOCUS FOR THE NEXT TWO WEEKS WILL BE RECOGNIZING WHEN WE ARE BEGINNING TO GET FULL AND STOPPING BEFORE FEELING OVERLY FULL. THE GOAL IS TO EAT JUST ENOUGH. WE WANT TO BE EATING SLOWLY AND FOCUSING ON OUR MEAL SO THAT WE CAN FEEL THE FULLNESS CUE COME ON. CHAPTER TWO HAS WAYS TO SLOW DOWN WHILE EATING SO YOU DON'T BLOW PAST NOTICING THE FULL FEELING.

WHEN WORKING WITH FULLNESS, I LIKE TO THINK OF IT ON A SCALE OF 0-10. ON THIS SCALE, 0 IS EQUAL TO NO FOOD IN YOUR STOMACH, VERY HUNGRY. AT THE OTHER END OF THE SCALE, 10 IS STUFFED, UNCOMFORTABLE, UNBUTTON PANTS AND LAY ON THE COUCH. OUR GOAL AT EACH MEAL IS TO GET TO AROUND 7 AND STOP. EATING TO THE FULLNESS POINT OF A 7 IS JUST ENOUGH. WE WANT TO BE ABLE TO COMFORTABLY MOVE AROUND YET BE CONTENT AFTER MEALS. BEING AT A 7 ON THE FULLNESS SCALE WOULD ALLOW YOU TO TAKE A WALK AFTER A MEAL. ANYTHING MORE THAN 7 CAN RESULT IN SLUGGISHNESS AND THAT OVERLY FULL, STRETCHED FEELING THAT IS NOT COMFORTABLE.

WHEN WORKING WITH THIS HABIT THERE ARE SEVERAL BAD HABITS THAT WE BEGIN TO NOTICE WE DO AND WE NEED TO WORK AROUND THOSE. WE BEGIN TO REALIZE THAT WE HAVE BEEN TRAINED TO CLEAN OUR PLATE AND WE WILL AT ALL COSTS. EVEN IF THAT MEANS BEING UNCOMFORTABLY FULL. THIS WILL TAKE PRACTICE BUT IT IS PERFECTLY OK TO LEAVE FOOD ON YOUR PLATE. IT IS IMPORTANT TO LISTEN TO YOUR BODY AND NOT STUFF IN THOSE LAST COUPLE BITES. A FEW BITES GOING INTO THE TRASH CAN SERVE YOUR BODY AND WEIGHT LOSS GOALS MUCH BETTER THAN THOSE BITES GOING INTO YOUR MOUTH. YOU ARE NO LONGER A MEMBER OF THE CLEAN PLATE CLUB! PRACTICE EACH MEAL LEAVING A FEW BITES ON YOUR PLATE IN ORDER TO STOP AT A FULLNESS LEVEL OF 7. EATING THOSE EXTRA BITES CAN PUT YOU OVER THE FULLNESS POINT AND AWAY FROM YOUR WEIGHT LOSS GOALS.

THE OTHER IMPORTANT THING TO REMEMBER IS THAT WE CAN HAVE FOOD ANYTIME WE ARE HUNGRY! HUNGER WILL ALWAYS COME BACK AND GIVE US THE OPPORTUNITY TO ENJOY FOOD ONCE AGAIN. NOW THAT WE KNOW WE CAN GET MORE LATER, WE DON'T HAVE TO EAT IT ALL AND GO PAST OUR FULLNESS POINT OF 7. BECAUSE THERE'S A MILLION MORE CHANCES!

OUR MINDSET TENDS TO GO TO "MUST EAT ALL NOW" BECAUSE OF CLEAN PLATE TRAINING. BUT THIS IS A SCARCITY MINDSET AROUND FOOD THAT WE DON'T NEED ANYMORE. WE LIVE IN A FOOD ABUNDANT WORLD. WE CAN GO TO A DRIVE THROUGH, GROCERY STORE, OR EVEN HAVE FOOD DELIVERED TO OUR DOOR WITHIN A FEW HOURS OF ORDERING! THERE'S ALWAYS MORE! FOOD IS ALWAYS AVAILABLE. WE DON'T HAVE TO EAT IT ALL AT THIS MEAL.

YOU CAN PUT IT IN A CONTAINER FOR LATER IF YOU DON'T LIKE THE IDEA OF THROWING IT AWAY. SOMETHING THAT HELPED ME TO LEAVE SOME BITES ON MY PLATE WAS TO PUT THE PLATE ASIDE IN CASE I WANTED TO ENJOY MORE LATER. WITHIN AN HOUR OR SO, I GOT TIRED OF LOOKING AT THE PLATE ON THE COUNTER AND REALIZING THAT THE FOOD WASN'T GOING TO TASTE THE SAME SO I'D TRASH IT. I'D TELL MYSELF I DESERVE SOMETHING FRESHLY MADE AT MY NEXT MEAL. THAT PAUSE BEFORE IT WENT STRAIGHT INTO THE TRASH HELPED ME TO LEARN TO LEAVE BITES ON MY PLATE.

THERE WILL BE AN ASPECT OF YOU, I CALLED MINE IMPULSIVE IRMA, THAT WILL WANT YOU TO FINISH THE FOOD. HE/SHE/THEY WILL SAY, "OH C'MON, IT'S ONLY A FEW BITES", "WHAT CAN IT HURT", OR "YOU DESERVE THIS". I JUST CONSISTENTLY REMINDED IRMA THAT WE CAN HAVE MORE FOOD LATER, THAT LISTENING TO FULLNESS IS IMPORTANT AND IS A HABIT WE NEED TO MASTER IN ORDER TO MEET WEIGHT LOSS/MAINTENANCE GOALS.

THE THING ABOUT OVEREATING IS THAT THE FOOD GOING INTO YOUR BODY AFTER YOU'VE REACHED THE FULLNESS LEVEL OF 7 IS JUST AS MUCH OF A WASTE AS IT IS GOING INTO THE ACTUAL TRASH CAN. SERVE YOUR BODY AND LET IT GO INTO THE TRASH CAN, RATHER THAN INTO YOU TO BE STORED AS UNWANTED FAT. NO MEAL IS A ONE TIME THING. YOU CAN HAVE MORE LATER!

ONCE YOU HAVE REACHED THAT FULLNESS LEVEL OF 7, MOVE YOUR PLATE AWAY, YOU WON'T BE EATING ANYMORE OF IT. IF YOU ARE IN THE HABIT OF GOING SEARCHING FOR MORE FOOD AFTER A MEAL, TRY HAVING SPARKLING WATER OR A CUP OF TEA AFTER MEALS. THIS SIGNALS THE END OF THE MEAL AND LETS YOUR BODY KNOW THAT YOU ARE DONE EATING. THIS BECOMES A HABIT AND YOU'LL QUICKLY BEGIN REACHING FOR THAT LOW CALORIE DRINK AFTER EATING, INSTEAD OF MORE FOOD.

REPEAT AFTER ME... "I CAN HAVE MORE LATER". THIS IS SOMETHING YOU WILL HAVE TO REMIND YOURSELF FREQUENTLY IN ORDER TO KEEP FROM OVEREATING AND BECOME COMFORTABLE LEAVING FOOD ON YOUR PLATE.

KEEP UP THE REMINDERS AND SPEND THE NEXT 2 WEEKS WORKING ON EATING TO A FULLNESS LEVEL OF 7 AT ALL MEALS. THAT'S LOTS OF PRACTICE AT EATING JUST ENOUGH. EACH MEAL IS AN OPPORTUNITY TO INVESTIGATE WHAT IS AND ISN'T WORKING. PAY ATTENTION TO THE WAY YOU ARE AT MEALS. ARE YOU EATING TOO QUICKLY? ARE YOU EATING DISTRACTED? GO BACK TO THE CHAPTERS THAT DISCUSSED MINDFUL EATING AND WAYS TO REALLY FOCUS DURING MEALS! THIS IS PRACTICE TO CHANGE YOUR RELATIONSHIP WITH FOOD AND BODY! KEEP DOING THE WORK! YOU CAN DO THIS!

THIS WAS THE LAST HABIT CHAPTER. THE REST IS INFORMATIONAL AND SOME JOURNAL PROMPTS TO BRING AWARENESS TO YOUR RELATIONSHIP WITH FOOD AND BODY. THERE WILL BE 14 DAILY JOURNAL PAGES OF "EATING JUST ENOUGH" TO THAT FULLNESS POINT OF 7 ON THE SCALE. THE WEEKLY ONES ARE ADDED IN AFTER YOU HAVE DONE THE HABIT FOR A WEEK. IF YOU HAVEN'T ALREADY, READ THE FOLLOWING CHAPTERS AROUND OTHER HABITS TO INCORPORATE PLUS DO THE FOCUS TECHNIQUES AND BODY IMAGES ACTIVITIES IN THE APPENDICES.

YOU CAN FIND MORE DAILY JOURNAL PAGES IN APPENDIX C TO TRACK AND COMPLETE THE FULL 16 WEEKS OF HABITS FOR MINDFUL EATING WEIGHT LOSS.

DAILY JOURNAL

DATE

TO DO LIST:

WATER TRACKER   ○○○○○○○

MOVEMENT

MOOD TRACKER   ☹ ☹ ☺ ☺ ☺

TODAY I AM GRATEFUL FOR:

HOURS OF SLEEP:

1.

3-4 MEALS, NO SNACKING	YES/NO
HUNGER 30 MINUTES BEFORE BREAKFAST	YES/NO

2.

HUNGER 30 MIN BEFORE LUNCH	YES/NO
HUNGER 30 MIN BEFORE DINNER	YES/NO

DAILY AFFIRMATION:

AT ALL MEALS, EAT JUST ENOUGH   YES/NO

CRAVINGS AND MY REACTION TO THEM

DAILY FOOD OR BODY WIN

INTENTION SETTING FOR TOMORROW

DAILY JOURNAL

DATE

TO DO LIST:

WATER TRACKER ◊◊◊◊◊◊◊

MOVEMENT

MOOD TRACKER ☹ ☹ ☺ ☺ ☺

TODAY I AM GRATEFUL FOR:

HOURS OF SLEEP:

1.

3-4 MEALS, NO SNACKING	YES/NO
HUNGER 30 MINUTES BEFORE BREAKFAST	YES/NO
HUNGER 30 MIN BEFORE LUNCH	YES/NO
HUNGER 30 MIN BEFORE DINNER	YES/NO
AT ALL MEALS, EAT JUST ENOUGH	YES/NO

2.

DAILY AFFIRMATION:

CRAVINGS AND MY REACTION TO THEM

DAILY FOOD OR BODY WIN

INTENTION SETTING FOR TOMORROW

DAILY JOURNAL

DATE

TO DO LIST:

_____

_____

_____

TODAY I AM GRATEFUL FOR:

1. _____

_____

2. _____

_____

DAILY AFFIRMATION:

_____

CRAVINGS AND MY REACTION TO THEM

_____

_____

_____

_____

INTENTION SETTING FOR TOMORROW

_____

_____

_____

WATER TRACKER ⬡⬡⬡⬡⬡⬡⬡

MOVEMENT

_____

_____

MOOD TRACKER ☹ ☹ 😐 ☺ 😊

HOURS OF SLEEP:

3-4 MEALS, NO SNACKING	YES/NO
HUNGER 30 MINUTES BEFORE BREAKFAST	YES/NO
HUNGER 30 MIN BEFORE LUNCH	YES/NO
HUNGER 30 MIN BEFORE DINNER	YES/NO
AT ALL MEALS, EAT JUST ENOUGH	YES/NO

DAILY FOOD OR BODY WIN

_____

_____

_____

DAILY JOURNAL

DATE

TO DO LIST:

_____

_____

_____

_____

TODAY I AM GRATEFUL FOR:

1.

_____

2.

_____

DAILY AFFIRMATION:

_____

CRAVINGS AND MY REACTION TO THEM

_____

_____

_____

_____

WATER TRACKER ◊◊◊◊◊◊◊

MOVEMENT

_____

MOOD TRACKER ☹ ☹ ☺ ☺ ☺

HOURS OF SLEEP:

3-4 MEALS, NO SNACKING	YES/NO
HUNGER 30 MINUTES BEFORE BREAKFAST	YES/NO
HUNGER 30 MIN BEFORE LUNCH	YES/NO
HUNGER 30 MIN BEFORE DINNER	YES/NO
AT ALL MEALS, EAT JUST ENOUGH	YES/NO

DAILY FOOD OR BODY WIN

_____

_____

_____

_____

INTENTION SETTING FOR TOMORROW

_____

_____

_____

DAILY JOURNAL

DATE

TO DO LIST:

_____

_____

_____

TODAY I AM GRATEFUL FOR:

1.

_____

2.

_____

DAILY AFFIRMATION:

_____

CRAVINGS AND MY REACTION TO THEM

_____

_____

_____

_____

WATER TRACKER   ⬡⬡⬡⬡⬡⬡⬡

MOVEMENT

_____

MOOD TRACKER   ☹ ☹ 😐 ☺ ☺

HOURS OF SLEEP:

3-4 MEALS, NO SNACKING   YES/NO

HUNGER 30 MINUTES BEFORE BREAKFAST   YES/NO

HUNGER 30 MIN BEFORE LUNCH   YES/NO

HUNGER 30 MIN BEFORE DINNER   YES/NO

AT ALL MEALS, EAT JUST ENOUGH   YES/NO

DAILY FOOD OR BODY WIN

_____

_____

_____

INTENTION SETTING FOR TOMORROW

_____

_____

_____

DAILY JOURNAL

DATE

TO DO LIST:

WATER TRACKER   ○○○○○○○

MOVEMENT

MOOD TRACKER   ☹ ☹ ☺ ☺ ☺

TODAY I AM GRATEFUL FOR:

HOURS OF SLEEP:

1.

3-4 MEALS, NO SNACKING	YES/NO
HUNGER 30 MINUTES BEFORE BREAKFAST	YES/NO
HUNGER 30 MIN BEFORE LUNCH	YES/NO
HUNGER 30 MIN BEFORE DINNER	YES/NO
AT ALL MEALS, EAT JUST ENOUGH	YES/NO

2.

DAILY AFFIRMATION:

CRAVINGS AND MY REACTION TO THEM

DAILY FOOD OR BODY WIN

INTENTION SETTING FOR TOMORROW

DAILY JOURNAL

DATE

TO DO LIST:

_____

_____

_____

TODAY I AM GRATEFUL FOR:

1. _____

_____

2. _____

_____

DAILY AFFIRMATION:

_____

CRAVINGS AND MY REACTION TO THEM

_____

_____

_____

_____

WATER TRACKER ◇◇◇◇◇◇◇

MOVEMENT

_____

MOOD TRACKER ☹ ☹ ☺ ☺ ☺

HOURS OF SLEEP:

3-4 MEALS, NO SNACKING   YES/NO

HUNGER 30 MINUTES BEFORE BREAKFAST   YES/NO

HUNGER 30 MIN BEFORE LUNCH   YES/NO

HUNGER 30 MIN BEFORE DINNER   YES/NO

AT ALL MEALS, EAT JUST ENOUGH   YES/NO

DAILY FOOD OR BODY WIN

_____

_____

_____

_____

INTENTION SETTING FOR TOMORROW

_____

_____

_____

WEEKLY JOURNAL

DATE

WEIGHT:

MY WHY...

_____

_____

_____

_____

WHAT IS GOING WELL WITH THIS WEEKS HABIT?

_____

_____

_____

WHAT COULD BE BETTER?

_____

_____

_____

GOALS FOR NEXT WEEK...

_____

_____

_____

DAILY JOURNAL

DATE

TO DO LIST:

TODAY I AM GRATEFUL FOR:

1.

2.

DAILY AFFIRMATION:

CRAVINGS AND MY REACTION TO THEM

WATER TRACKER   ○○○○○○○

MOVEMENT

MOOD TRACKER   ☹ ☹ ☺ ☺ ☺

HOURS OF SLEEP:

3-4 MEALS, NO SNACKING	YES/NO
HUNGER 30 MINUTES BEFORE BREAKFAST	YES/NO
HUNGER 30 MIN BEFORE LUNCH	YES/NO
HUNGER 30 MIN BEFORE DINNER	YES/NO
AT ALL MEALS, EAT JUST ENOUGH	YES/NO

DAILY FOOD OR BODY WIN

INTENTION SETTING FOR TOMORROW

DAILY JOURNAL

DATE

TO DO LIST:

WATER TRACKER ○○○○○○○

MOVEMENT

MOOD TRACKER ☹ ☹ ☺ ☺ ☺

TODAY I AM GRATEFUL FOR:

HOURS OF SLEEP:

1.

3-4 MEALS, NO SNACKING   YES/NO

HUNGER 30 MINUTES BEFORE BREAKFAST   YES/NO

2.

HUNGER 30 MIN BEFORE LUNCH   YES/NO

HUNGER 30 MIN BEFORE DINNER   YES/NO

DAILY AFFIRMATION:

AT ALL MEALS, EAT JUST ENOUGH   YES/NO

CRAVINGS AND MY REACTION TO THEM

DAILY FOOD OR BODY WIN

INTENTION SETTING FOR TOMORROW

DAILY JOURNAL

DATE

TO DO LIST:

_____

_____

_____

TODAY I AM GRATEFUL FOR:

1.
_____

2.
_____

DAILY AFFIRMATION:

_____

CRAVINGS AND MY REACTION TO THEM

_____

_____

_____

_____

WATER TRACKER ⬡⬡⬡⬡⬡⬡⬡

MOVEMENT

_____

MOOD TRACKER ☹ ☹ ☺ ☺ ☺

HOURS OF SLEEP:

3-4 MEALS, NO SNACKING	YES/NO
HUNGER 30 MINUTES BEFORE BREAKFAST	YES/NO
HUNGER 30 MIN BEFORE LUNCH	YES/NO
HUNGER 30 MIN BEFORE DINNER	YES/NO
AT ALL MEALS, EAT JUST ENOUGH	YES/NO

DAILY FOOD OR BODY WIN

_____

_____

_____

_____

INTENTION SETTING FOR TOMORROW

_____

_____

_____

DAILY JOURNAL

DATE

TO DO LIST:

_____

_____

_____

WATER TRACKER   ◌◌◌◌◌◌◌

MOVEMENT

_____

_____

MOOD TRACKER   ☹ ☹ ☺ ☺ ☺

TODAY I AM GRATEFUL FOR:

1. _____

2. _____

DAILY AFFIRMATION:

_____

HOURS OF SLEEP:

3-4 MEALS, NO SNACKING	YES/NO
HUNGER 30 MINUTES BEFORE BREAKFAST	YES/NO
HUNGER 30 MIN BEFORE LUNCH	YES/NO
HUNGER 30 MIN BEFORE DINNER	YES/NO
AT ALL MEALS, EAT JUST ENOUGH	YES/NO

CRAVINGS AND MY REACTION TO THEM

_____

_____

_____

_____

DAILY FOOD OR BODY WIN

_____

_____

_____

_____

INTENTION SETTING FOR TOMORROW

_____

_____

_____

DAILY JOURNAL

DATE

TO DO LIST:

_____

_____

_____

TODAY I AM GRATEFUL FOR:

1. _____

_____

2. _____

_____

DAILY AFFIRMATION:

_____

CRAVINGS AND MY REACTION TO THEM

_____

_____

_____

_____

WATER TRACKER ◇◇◇◇◇◇◇

MOVEMENT

_____

MOOD TRACKER ☹ ☹ ☺ ☺ ☺

HOURS OF SLEEP:

3-4 MEALS, NO SNACKING	YES/NO
HUNGER 30 MINUTES BEFORE BREAKFAST	YES/NO
HUNGER 30 MIN BEFORE LUNCH	YES/NO
HUNGER 30 MIN BEFORE DINNER	YES/NO
AT ALL MEALS, EAT JUST ENOUGH	YES/NO

DAILY FOOD OR BODY WIN

_____

_____

_____

_____

INTENTION SETTING FOR TOMORROW

_____

_____

_____

DAILY JOURNAL

DATE

TO DO LIST:

WATER TRACKER ○○○○○○○

MOVEMENT

TODAY I AM GRATEFUL FOR:

MOOD TRACKER ☹ ☹ ☺ ☺ ☺

HOURS OF SLEEP:

1.

3-4 MEALS, NO SNACKING	YES/NO

HUNGER 30 MINUTES BEFORE BREAKFAST	YES/NO

2.

HUNGER 30 MIN BEFORE LUNCH	YES/NO

HUNGER 30 MIN BEFORE DINNER	YES/NO

DAILY AFFIRMATION:

AT ALL MEALS, EAT JUST ENOUGH	YES/NO

CRAVINGS AND MY REACTION TO THEM

DAILY FOOD OR BODY WIN

INTENTION SETTING FOR TOMORROW

DAILY JOURNAL

DATE

TO DO LIST:

WATER TRACKER ◇◇◇◇◇◇◇

MOVEMENT

MOOD TRACKER ☹ ☹ 😐 ☺ 😊

TODAY I AM GRATEFUL FOR:

HOURS OF SLEEP:

1.

3-4 MEALS, NO SNACKING	YES/NO
HUNGER 30 MINUTES BEFORE BREAKFAST	YES/NO
HUNGER 30 MIN BEFORE LUNCH	YES/NO
HUNGER 30 MIN BEFORE DINNER	YES/NO
AT ALL MEALS, EAT JUST ENOUGH	YES/NO

2.

DAILY AFFIRMATION:

CRAVINGS AND MY REACTION TO THEM

DAILY FOOD OR BODY WIN

INTENTION SETTING FOR TOMORROW

WEEKLY JOURNAL

WEIGHT:

MY WHY...
_____
_____
_____
_____

WHAT IS GOING WELL WITH THIS WEEKS HABIT?
_____
_____
_____
_____

WHAT COULD BE BETTER?
_____
_____
_____
_____

GOALS FOR NEXT WEEK...
_____
_____
_____

_____
CONTINUE TO APPENDIX C FOR MORE DAILY, WEEKLY, AND MONTHLY JOURNAL
PAGES TO COMPLETE THE ENTIRE 16 WEEKS OF HABIT SUCCESS

CHAPTER 7
EMOTIONAL EATING

FOR SOME, FOOD FOR COMFORT HAS BECOME A LIFESTYLE. FEEL GOOD HORMONES IN OUR BRAINS ARE SECRETED WHEN WE HAVE CHOCOLATE, ICE CREAM, CHIPS AND OTHER TASTY TREATS. THESE FEEL GOOD HORMONES TEMPORARILY DIMINISH WHATEVER STRESS, FRUSTRATION, SADNESS, OR ANGER THAT WE HAVE. SO OF COURSE ANY TIME WE ARE TRIGGERED BY EMOTIONS WE REACH FOR COOKIES! WE CRAVE THE FEEL GOOD FEELING!

IF YOU ARE HAVING A TOUGH MEETING AT WORK OR ARGUING WITH YOUR SPOUSE AND YOUR HEAD IS SCREAMING FOR CHOCOLATE, COOKIES, AND CHIPS, THEN THAT IS AN EMOTIONAL EATING RESPONSE. FROM PREVIOUS CYCLES OF EMOTIONAL EATING, OUR BRAINS KNOW THE STRESS YOU ARE FEELING CAN BE ALLEVIATED BY THE SALTY AND SWEET PACKAGED FOODS. THE BRAIN AND BODY WANTS THESE LESS THAN FAVORABLE FEELINGS TO GO AWAY RIGHT NOW. THE QUICKEST ROUTE TO DITCH THE EMOTIONS IS BY HEADING TO THE PANTRY OR VENDING MACHINE. EACH INCIDENCE OF THIS MEANS WE ARE PROGRAMMING OUR BRAIN FOR SNACKING AND TURNING TO FOOD WHEN WE ARE STRESSED. IT MIGHT NOT EVEN BE A CONSCIOUS THOUGHT ANYMORE THAT YOU'RE STRUGGLING AND REACH FOR FOOD. YOU MIGHT JUST GO STRAIGHT TO THE FOOD, NO THOUGHT AT ALL AS TO WHAT'S GOING ON.

BECOMING AWARE OF YOUR EMOTIONS IS THE FIRST STEP TO ENDING EMOTIONAL EATING. TO BECOME AWARE OF HOW YOU'RE FEELING AT ANY TIME, YOU WILL BEGIN TO CHECK IN WITH YOURSELF. I RECOMMEND CHECKING IN WITH YOURSELF BEFORE MEALS OR SETTING A REMINDER ON YOUR PHONE TO GO OFF A FEW TIMES A DAY. IF DONE WITH MEALS, THIS GIVES YOU AT LEAST 3 OPPORTUNITIES A DAY TO INVESTIGATE YOUR EMOTIONAL STATE AND BECOME MORE AWARE OF WHAT YOU ARE FEELING THROUGHOUT THE DAY OR AS YOU START A MEAL.

SIMPLY ASK YOURSELF, "HOW AM I ACTUALLY FEELING?". WITHOUT USING JUST THE TERMS GOOD OR BAD TO DESCRIBE YOUR EMOTIONS. NOTICE EVEN THE SMALLEST HINT OF FRUSTRATION, ANGER, SADNESS, CONTENTMENT, HAPPINESS OR EXCITEMENT. ONCE YOU'VE NAMED THE EMOTION YOU ARE EXPERIENCING, YOU CAN GO FURTHER AND TRY TO FIGURE OUT WHY YOU ARE FEELING THIS WAY. HAS WORK BEEN EXCEPTIONALLY GOOD TODAY? DID KAREN SAY SOMETHING YOU DIDN'T AGREE WITH AND THAT HAS STAYED WITH YOU? GET TO KNOW YOUR FEELINGS AND WHAT IS CAUSING THEM.

BY TAKING THE TIME TO INVESTIGATE THE WAY YOU FEEL RANDOMLY THROUGHOUT THE DAY YOU BEGIN TO FLEX THAT EMOTIONAL AWARENESS MUSCLE. YOU BEGIN TO BE ABLE TO SAY "I'M FEELING ___ AND THIS IS WHY". WHEN YOU NAME THE EMOTION AND WHAT'S CAUSING IT, YOU DO TWO THINGS:

1) TAKING A PAUSE TO NOTICE THE EMOTION MEANS THAT YOU AREN'T HEADING STRAIGHT FOR FOOD AND CAN CHOOSE TO DO SOMETHING ELSE INSTEAD, AND
2) NAMING THE EMOTION TENDS TO WEAKEN IT'S HOLD ON YOU.

YOU ARE ABLE TO LET IT GO AND MOVE ON BECAUSE YOU HAVE NOTICED IT. BEING ABLE TO SAY "I'M MAD BECAUSE TIMMY CALLED ME A SELF CENTERED KNOW-IT-ALL", TAKES THE PRESSURE OFF THE SITUATION. IT RELEASES THAT MADNESS VALVE SIMPLY BY NOTICING IT. WITHOUT NAMING IT, THE EMOTION JUST BREWS AND GROWS AS YOU STEW ABOUT THE EXPERIENCE.

MY GOAL WITH THIS INFORMATION IS TO GET THE EMOTIONAL EATING TO STOP. TO REPROGRAM YOUR BRAIN TO FIND OTHER THINGS THAT ARE FULFILLING WHEN YOU HAVE AN EMOTIONAL NEED, INSTEAD OF EATING. BECAUSE WE KNOW THE DOWNSIDES OF CONTINUING TO EAT TO SATISFY EMOTIONS. WE DON'T LIKE THE WAY WE FEEL AFTER. WE HAVE THE GUILT OF "I DID IT AGAIN" OR "WHY AM I SO OUT OF CONTROL AROUND FOOD". ALSO EMOTIONAL EATING IS PART OF THE REASON WE ARE CARRYING EXTRA WEIGHT AROUND, SINCE WE ARE PROVIDING OUR BODY WITH MORE NUTRIENTS THAN IT NEEDS.

YOU KNOW THIS IS NOT THE RELATIONSHIP YOU WANT WITH FOOD BUT THE EMOTIONAL EATING CYCLE IS REPETITIVE. IT CAN ALSO BE CHALLENGING TO CONVINCE OUR BRAINS THAT THERE ARE OTHER SOOTHING ACTIVITIES. THE FIRST STEP IS TO NOTICE YOU ARE EXPERIENCING AN EMOTION. AS YOU GET IN THE HABIT OF THIS FROM THE ABOVE MENTIONED CHECK IN, YOU WILL GET FAMILIAR WITH WHEN YOU ARE FEELING SOMETHING. IF THIS FEELING IS FOLLOWED BY A DESIRE TO EAT, INVESTIGATE FURTHER. WHEN WAS THE LAST TIME I ATE? SHOULD I BE HUNGRY RIGHT NOW? AM I HUNGRY FOR ONLY ONE FOOD (PROBABLY SOMETHING SWEET OR SALTY IN A PACKAGE) OR WOULD I HAVE AN APPLE OR SOME BROCCOLI?

ONCE YOU HAVE DETERMINED THAT YOU ARE NOT ACTUALLY HUNGRY AND YOU ARE SEEKING THE COMFORT THAT FOOD PROVIDES, YOU CAN BEGIN TO LOOK FOR OTHER THINGS THAT WILL BRING HAPPINESS. BEFORE DOING ANYTHING ELSE TO RELEASE THE EMOTION OR SEEKING OTHER COMFORT, I WOULD SUGGEST DISTANCING YOURSELF FROM THE FOOD. GO TO THE OTHER END OF THE HOUSE, TO ANOTHER ROOM, OR OUTSIDE. GIVING YOURSELF THAT SPACE FROM THE SNACKS DIMINISHES THE IMPULSE. THIS THEN MAKES IT EASIER TO FIND SOMETHING ELSE TO APPEASE.

THERE ARE A NUMBER OF THINGS TO TRY INSTEAD OF EATING. PHYSICAL MOVEMENT CAN HELP TO MOVE THE EMOTION THROUGH YOUR BODY. IT CAN HELP TO RELEASE THE EMOTION SO YOU AREN'T STUCK IN AN UNFAVORABLE FEELING AND WANTING FOOD. WALK, TURN ON A GOOD SONG AND DANCE, RUN, SHAKE (DESCRIBED BELOW), STRETCH, ANY KIND OF MOVEMENT YOU LIKE. MOVEMENT CAN BE USED IN AS SHORT A TIME AS A QUICK TRIP TO THE BATHROOM IF YOU'RE AT WORK OR IT CAN BE AS LONG AS A WALK OUTSIDE IF YOU'RE HOME. JUST MOVE YOUR BODY!

IF YOU HAVE A SHORT AMOUNT OF TIME OR ARE AT WORK AND DON'T HAVE MUCH SPACE, TRY SHAKING. SHAKING HAS A WONDERFUL WAY OF GETTING YOUR MIND OFF OF WHAT'S BOTHERING YOU.

IT REQUIRES SOME EFFORT AND ONCE YOU'VE CEASED THE EFFORT YOU REALLY GET TO RELAX AND IT FEELS GOOD! IT IS LIKE AN ESCAPE BUTTON FOR YOUR BRAIN. DO IT AS MANY TIMES IN A ROW AS YOU NEED TO SHIFT OUT OF THE EMOTION YOU ARE EXPERIENCING.

TO DO THE SHAKING TECHNIQUE, SET A TIMER FOR 30-45 SECONDS. UNTIL THE TIMER GOES OFF, SHAKE YOUR ENTIRE BODY, LIKE A DOG OUT OF THE BATH. SHAKE ARMS, LEGS, SHOULDERS, HIPS, EVERYTHING! YOU CAN EVEN VISUALIZE THE NEGATIVE FEELINGS SHAKING OFF OF YOU, COMING OUT OF YOUR FINGERTIPS AS YOU FLICK THEM LIKE YOU'VE JUST WASHED YOUR HANDS. THIS WILL GET YOUR HEART RATE UP QUICKLY AND ALLOW UNPLEASANT FEELINGS TO DISSIPATE. YOU MIGHT EVEN LAUGH AT YOURSELF FOR DOING SOMETHING SO SILLY BUT YOU DEFINITELY WON'T BE REACHING FOR FOOD AFTER COMPLETING THIS EXERCISE.

THERE ARE OTHER THINGS THAT BRING PEACE DEPENDING ON WHETHER YOU ARE AT HOME OR WORK. YOU COULD GET A HUG FROM A FAMILY MEMBER, PET AN ANIMAL, GO OUTSIDE FOR SOME FRESH AIR, GRAB A SOFT BLANKET, HAVE A WARM CUP OF TEA, OR TAKE A BATHROOM BREAK FOR SOME DEEP BREATHS. I LIKE TO USE THE MICROWAVABLE SHOULDER WRAP OR WARM COMPRESSES THAT YOU CAN BUY ONLINE FOR THE CONTENTMENT AND SOOTHING WARMTH THEY BRING. CHECK OUT APPENDIX B IN THIS JOURNAL FOR BREATHING AND FOCUSING TECHNIQUES THAT CAN BE DONE AS WELL TO AVOID EMOTIONAL EATING.

REPEAT ANY OF THESE TECHNIQUES AS MANY TIMES AS NEEDED. CONTINUE TO REACH FOR SOMETHING THAT BRINGS JOY OTHER THAN FOOD. FIND WHAT YOU LIKE AND STICK TO IT. YOU HAVE TO REMEMBER THAT EACH TIME YOU CHOOSE SOMETHING ELSE OVER EMOTIONAL EATING YOU ARE TEARING AWAY AT THAT OLD PROGRAM IN YOUR BRAIN AND INSTALLING A NEW ONE THAT CHANGES THE WAY YOU ARE WITH FOOD. THIS IS CHALLENGING WORK BUT OH SO WORTH IT! BE PROUD OF YOURSELF WHEN YOU'VE TAKEN THE TIME AND EFFORT TO NOT EMOTIONAL EAT AND WRITE IT ON YOUR DAILY JOURNAL PAGE. IF YOU GO AHEAD AND HAVE THE COOKIES IN A FEW SITUATIONS, KNOW THAT THIS CHANGE TAKES TIME AND THERE WILL BE OTHER CHANCES FOR SUCCESS. WRITE ON YOUR DAILY JOURNAL PAGE WHAT DID OR DIDN'T WORK AND GIVE YOURSELF SOME GRACE AS YOU CHANGE THE WAY YOU INTERACT WITH FOOD.

EMOTIONAL EATING CAN FALL INTO THE "CRAVINGS" CATEGORY. BE SURE TO USE THE "CRAVINGS + REACTION" SECTION ON YOUR DAILY JOURNAL SHEETS TO RECORD HOW YOU ARE NAVIGATING FOOD DESIRES WHEN NOT HUNGRY.

YOU'VE NOW LEARNED ABOUT EMOTIONAL EATING AND ITS EFFECTS. ALONG WITH THE HABITS OF EATING 3-4 MEALS PER DAY AND RECOGNIZING HUNGER/FULLNESS. ALL THESE HABITS WILL CREATE TRUE CHANGE. KEEP TAKING THE TIME EACH DAY TO CHECK OFF YOUR ACCOMPLISHMENTS AND SHOW UP FOR YOURSELF! ON TO CHAPTER 8!

CHAPTER 8
STOP THE DIETING CYCLE

IN ORDER TO HAVE A NATURAL RELATIONSHIP WITH FOOD, DIETING HAS TO GO. DIETS ARE NOT SUSTAINABLE. YOU DO NOT WANT TO HAVE TO COUNT EVERYTHING THAT YOU EAT OR LEAVE OUT ENTIRE FOOD GROUPS FOR THE REST OF YOUR LIFE, IN ORDER TO MAINTAIN OR LOSE WEIGHT. YES, DIETS MAY WORK IN THE SHORT TERM BUT WE ALMOST ALWAYS STOP DIETING AND RETURN TO OUR NORMAL HABITS AROUND EATING WHICH RESULTS IN WEIGHT GAIN. OUR NORMAL WAY OF EATING WHEN NOT ON A DIET IS DISREGARDING OUR HUNGER AND FULLNESS PLUS BINGE EATING AND/OR EMOTIONAL EATING. ALL A RECIPE FOR GAINING BACK THE WEIGHT WE'VE LOST AND MORE. BY USING THE HABITS FROM THE PREVIOUS CHAPTERS, YOU CHANGE THE WAY YOU INTERACT WITH FOOD AND IF DONE CONSISTENTLY CAN RESULT IN BODY CHANGE AS WELL.

WHEN WE ARE ON A DIET, WE ARE RESTRICTING FOOD GROUPS AND CALORIE INTAKE. IF WE THINK BACK TO THE EARLY TIMES OF MAN, THERE WAS FOOD SCARCITY. WHEN WE ACTUALLY HAD TO HUNT, GROW, AND COOK ALL FOOD WITH NO EXCEPTIONS. WHEN WE RESTRICT INTAKE OUR BRAINS REVERT BACK TO THAT EARLY PROGRAMMING THAT IS WORRIED ABOUT SURVIVAL DURING A FAMINE. OUR BRAIN AND BODY'S THINK THERE IS NOT ENOUGH FOOD. WE NEED MORE INTAKE TO STAY ALIVE. MUST EAT LOTS NOW! SO WHEN AT THE END OF THE DAY/WEEK/MONTH, WHEN YOU FEEL YOU CAN'T CONTROL YOURSELF AROUND FOOD ANYMORE, IT'S BECAUSE YOU'VE PUT YOUR BRAIN AND BODY IN THAT FAMINE STATE. THE DIET IS THE FAILURE, NOT YOU. WE WEREN'T MEANT TO ALWAYS BE IN A STATE OF RESTRICTION OR FAMINE.

WHEN YOU LISTEN TO YOUR BODY AROUND HUNGER AND FULLNESS AND LOSE THE RESTRICTING THEN OVEREATING CYCLE, LIFE GETS EASIER! YOU GET TO ENJOY ALL THE FOOD! EVEN A BURGER AND FRENCH FRIES WITHOUT THE SUSPECTED WEIGHT GAIN BECAUSE YOU KNOW THAT YOUR BODY WILL LET YOU KNOW WHEN ALL THAT NUTRITION IS USED UP AND IT'S TIME FOR MORE.

YOU JUST HAVE TO LEARN TO ALLOW! ALLOW YOURSELF TO HAVE ALL THINGS WITHOUT JUDGMENT. TO HAVE NO FOOD BE ON A PEDESTAL, YOU COULD TAKE IT OR LEAVE IT. IN THE FOLLOWING JOURNAL PAGES IS AN "OFF LIMITS FOODS" SHEET TO FILL OUT. THIS IS THE STUFF YOU DON'T ALLOW IN THE HOUSE OR THAT YOU CAN'T CONTROL YOURSELF AROUND WHEN IT'S AVAILABLE. THIS LIST SHOWS YOU THE FOODS YOU HAVE PLACED ON A PEDESTAL. ANY FOOD ON A PEDESTAL GETS MORE ENERGY AND ATTENTION THAT IT NEEDS. WE WILL BEGIN TAKING FOOD OFF THE PEDESTAL AND EVERYTHING WILL BECOME NEUTRAL BY GRANTING YOURSELF ACCESS TO THEM ONCE AGAIN.

YOU WILL BEGIN DETHRONING THESE FOODS BY INCORPORATING THEM INTO YOUR MEALS. THEY WILL BE EATEN PLATED AND MINDFULLY SO YOU CAN TRULY ENJOY THEM. EVEN DESSERTS WILL BE ON YOUR PLATE TO BE SAVORED WITH EVERYTHING ELSE! I CAME TO FIND THAT WHEN I WASN'T EATING THINGS VERY QUICKLY IN THE PANTRY THAT THEY WEREN'T AS ENJOYABLE AS THEY ONCE WERE. AS I TOOK THE THRILL AWAY AND REALIZED I COULD HAVE THEM WITH A MEAL WHENEVER I WANTED, THEY LOST THEIR CHARM. I COULD TAKE IT OR LEAVE IT.

SINCE THESE ITEMS CAN TRIGGER THOUGHTS, BELIEFS, FEELINGS OR ACTIONS IN RELATION TO THEM, WE CAN ALSO CALL THESE OFF LIMIT FOODS BY THE NAME OF TRIGGER FOODS. I RECOMMEND STAYING ON ONE TRIGGER FOOD UNTIL IT'S LESS APPEALING. ONCE YOU CAN TAKE IT OR LEAVE IT, IT'S TIME TO MOVE ON TO THE NEXT ONE. HAVE THESE FOODS AT ANY MEAL YOU WANT! THIS IS YOUR PERMISSION SLIP TO HAVE THE DELICIOUS FOOD YOU HAVE JUDGED AND HAVEN'T ALLOWED YOURSELF TO ENJOY. HAVE THESE DELIGHTFUL THINGS FEELING GRATITUDE FOR THE FOOD ITSELF AND YOUR BODY'S ABILITY TO DIGEST IT WITHOUT WEIGHT GAIN.

SOME PEOPLE HAVE EXPRESSED CONCERN FOR WEIGHT GAIN WHEN ALLOWING "OFF LIMIT" FOODS. THEY SAY IF I ALLOW MYSELF TO HAVE THEM I WON'T STOP! MY ANSWER IS ALWAYS YOU MIGHT NOT BE ABLE TO STOP AT FIRST... BECAUSE YOU NEVER ALLOW THEM, YOUR BRAIN IS GOING TO HAVE A HARD TIME TRUSTING THAT YOU WON'T PUT THEM BACK ON THE PEDESTAL. WHICH MEANS TAKING THEM AWAY AGAIN. WITH EACH EXPERIENCE THAT YOU ALLOW THESE FOODS, YOUR BRAIN BEGINS TO TRUST THAT YOU'LL HAVE ANOTHER CHANCE TO EAT IT, SO IT'S SAFE TO STOP AT CONTENT AND NOT BINGE. IT'S ALL PRACTICE. IT WILL BECOME MORE NATURAL AS YOU KEEP AT IT. JUST REMEMBER THE MANTRA, "I CAN HAVE MORE LATER" AND CONTINUE MAKING ALL FOOD NEUTRAL.

THE OTHER ABSOLUTE KEY TO ENJOYING ANY AND ALL FOODS IS TO PAY ATTENTION TO HUNGER AND FULLNESS. EVEN IF YOU HAVE CAKE, FRENCH FRIES, AND PIZZA, YOUR BODY WILL DIGEST IT PROPERLY WITHOUT LEADING TO WEIGHT GAIN IF YOU ARE REFRAINING FROM EATING UNTIL YOU ARE HUNGRY AGAIN. YOU WILL START TO NOTICE THAT HEAVIER MEALS MAY TAKE 5-6 HOURS UNTIL YOU GET HUNGRY AGAIN COMPARED TO THE NORMAL 3-4 WITH A TYPICAL MEAL. AND THAT'S OKAY! SOME THINGS DO TAKE LONGER TO DIGEST. TRUST THAT YOUR BODY KNOWS WHAT IT IS DOING.

AS YOU ADD IN YOUR OFF LIMIT FOODS, WATCH THE NEGATIVE THOUGHTS OF "THIS IS GOING STRAIGHT TO MY THIGHS" OR "THE SCALE WILL REFLECT THIS TOMORROW". REMEMBER THE BODY ACHIEVES WHAT THE MIND BELIEVES. SO BE SURE TO INSTALL THE PROGRAMMING OF HOW YOU WANT YOUR BODY TO WORK FOR YOU! TRY SAYING "THANK YOU BODY FOR DIGESTING THIS MEAL APPROPRIATELY AND NOT ADDING EXTRA WEIGHT". OR "I TRUST MY BODY'S SIGNALS OF HUNGER AND FULLNESS TO CUE ME WHEN TO EAT AGAIN." THIS WAY OF LIFE ALLOWS YOU TO TRUST YOUR BODY AND HAVE ALL THINGS.

ANOTHER TRICK TO TRY WITH DESSERTS OR OTHER FOODS IS TO START HAVING A MINDSET THAT IF YOU'RE GOING TO HAVE IT, IT'S GOT TO BE THE BEST. DON'T SETTLE FOR OFF BRAND COOKIES FROM THE PANTRY THAT ARE JUST OK. IF YOU WANT COOKIES, BAKE THEM FROM SCRATCH OR MAKE THE CONSCIOUS EFFORT TO STOP BY THE LOCAL BAKERY. SAME GOES FOR DAY-OLD CAKE LEFTOVERS IN THE OFFICE. IF IT'S NOT THE BEST AT THIS POINT, DON'T HAVE IT AND SEEK OUT WHAT YOU ACTUALLY DESERVE. WHICH IS SOMETHING FRESH AND SUPER TASTY. WE TEND TO HAVE THINGS JUST BECAUSE THEY ARE AROUND OR BECAUSE THEY ARE OFFERED BUT WE CAN CERTAINLY TURN THEM DOWN WITH A POLITE NO THANK YOU TO HAVE THE PERFECT VERSION LATER OR WHEN WE ARE HUNGRY AGAIN. FOOD IS ALWAYS AVAILABLE AND OUR MAGNIFICENT BODY'S ARE WORTHY OF THE GOOD STUFF!

ANOTHER JOURNAL PAGE YOU WILL FIND IN THE NEXT FEW PAGES IS THE GOOD VS BAD FOODS SHEET. THIS SHEET HELPS YOU GET VERY CLEAR ON THE FOODS THAT ARE STILL ON A PEDESTAL OR HAVE POWER IN YOUR MIND. CHALLENGE YOUR THINKING AROUND FOOD. WHAT FOODS DO YOU JUDGE OTHERS FOR EATING? WHAT FOODS DO YOU THINK NEGATIVELY ABOUT WHEN YOU'RE EATING THEM?

WHEN I SAW MY FRIENDS EATING FRENCH FRIES, I WOULD POLITELY DECLINE THEM AND I WOULD REMARK TO MYSELF "I JUST DON'T EAT LIKE THAT". BUT IN REALITY I WOULDN'T ALLOW MYSELF TO HAVE FRIES BECAUSE I DEEMED THEM AS "BAD". THEREFORE THEY NEEDED TO BE TAKEN OFF THE PEDESTAL.
I HAD WORK TO DO AROUND FRENCH FRIES, SO I SET OUT TO EAT THEM MINDFULLY AND WITHOUT JUDGMENT. BEFORE LONG I WAS NO LONGER JUDGING MYSELF OR OTHERS FOR ENJOYING FRIES AND OTHER FOODS.

ASK YOURSELF IS THE FOOD LISTED IN THE "BAD" CATEGORY ACTUALLY "BAD"? CAN A BROWNIE BE COMPARED TO HITLER? NOPE! SOME FOODS ARE MORE NUTRIENT DENSE THAN OTHERS, SURE, BUT WILL HAVING A BROWNIE SET YOU UP TO GO TO PRISON FOR LIFE? NO! FOOD IS NOT A MORAL ISSUE. THERE IS NO GOOD OR BAD FOOD. THE LESS YOU JUDGE FOOD THE MORE YOU ARE ABLE TO TAKE BACK THE POWER FROM IT. TAKING THE JUDGMENT OUT MAKES IT POSSIBLE TO ENJOY ALL FOODS WITHOUT THINKING TWICE ABOUT IT. THAT'S THE WAY YOU WANT YOUR RELATIONSHIP WITH FOOD TO BE! ATTEMPT TO CHANGE YOUR VERBIAGE AT MEALS. THINK OF SOMETHING AS "HAVING LESS NUTRIENTS" IN THE PLACE OF "BAD" OR THINK OF IT AS NOT SERVING YOUR BODY AS MUCH AS OTHER MORE NOURISHING FOODS CAN. IT'S ALL HOW YOU HAVE IT IN YOUR MIND.

OFF LIMITS FOOD

DATE

LIST THE FOODS BELOW YOU CAN'T CONTROL YOURSELF AROUND, THAT YOU CAN'T HAVE IN THE HOUSE, OR THE STUFF YOU NEVER BUY BUT THINK ABOUT FREQUENTLY. ADD FOOD ANYTIME YOU ARE REMINDED OF THEM.

_____

EX: COOKIES, BROWNIES, POTATO CHIPS, ETC

_____

_____

_____

_____

_____

_____

_____

_____

_____

_____

_____

_____

_____

THIS LIST SHOWS THE FOODS YOU HAVE PLACED ON A PEDESTAL AND WON'T ALLOW YOURSELF TO HAVE. IN LETTING GO OF THE DIETING/RESTRICTING, YOU WILL ADD THIS LIST OF FOODS TO "CAN HAVE" AS LONG AS THEY ARE EATEN SLOWLY AND MINDFULLY. CHIPPING AWAY AT THESE FOODS ONE BY ONE WILL NORMALIZE ALL FOODS AND YOU WILL NO LONGER BE OUT OF CONTROL AROUND THEM BECAUSE YOU KNOW YOU CAN HAVE THEM WHENEVER. NOW GET TO WORK ACTUALLY ENJOYING FOODS YOU DON'T NORMALLY ALLOW YOURSELF TO!

GOOD VS BAD FOODS

DATE

THIS LIST HELPS YOU TO NOTICE HOW MUCH YOU JUDGE FOOD. YES SOME FOODS HAVE MORE NUTRIENTS THAN OTHERS BUT FOOD IS NOT A MORAL ISSUE. IT'S JUST FOOD! CHANGING YOUR VIEW POINT CAN HELP TO HAVE A MORE NATURAL RELATIONSHIP WITH FOOD.

GOOD FOODS: EX-SALAD

_____

_____

_____

_____

_____

_____

_____

_____

BAD FOODS: EX- FRENCH FRIES

_____

_____

_____

_____

_____

_____

_____

CHAPTER 9
WATER AND SLEEP

THE AMOUNT OF WATER AND SLEEP YOU GET CAN AFFECT YOUR SUCCESS. BEING SURE TO INCLUDE THESE TWO HABITS IN YOUR DAILY ROUTINE WILL PUT YOU AT AN ADVANTAGE TO REACH YOUR GOALS.

WATER IS SO VERY IMPORTANT! OUR BODIES ARE 60% WATER. THE MORE HYDRATED WE ARE, THE MORE EFFICIENTLY OUR BODIES CAN FUNCTION. THERE CAN EVEN BE TIMES WHEN THIRST IS MISTAKEN FOR HUNGER SO WE GRAB FOR FOOD WHEN REALLY WE JUST NEED A GLASS OF WATER. STAYING HYDRATED WITH AT LEAST 8 GLASSES OR 64 OUNCES OF WATER EACH DAY CAN HELP AVOID THIS. SO THE NEXT TIME YOU GRAB A DRINK, PUT DOWN THE SODA OR JUICE AND DRINK SOME WATER!

SLEEP IS THE OTHER KEY TO MAINTAINING HEALTHY HABITS. WHEN YOU ARE SLEEP DEPRIVED EVERYTHING IS AFFECTED. YOU MIGHT BE TEMPTED TO LOAD UP ON SUGARY FOODS AND HIGH CALORIE COFFEES FOR ENERGY. YOU MIGHT SKIP YOUR WORKOUT OR ABANDON COOKING SOMETHING NOURISHING AT HOME TO HIT UP A DRIVE THROUGH INSTEAD. ALL IN THE NAME OF BEING FATIGUED.

SO IN ORDER TO MAKE THE BEST CHOICES FOR YOURSELF AND YOUR BODY, MAKE SURE YOU ARE GETTING 7-9 HOURS OF SLEEP AT NIGHT. CREATE A BEDTIME RITUAL THAT YOU DO CONSISTENTLY TO LET YOUR BODY KNOW IT'S TIME TO WIND DOWN. THIS RITUAL SHOULD NOT INCLUDE ELECTRONICS IN BED. THIS HAS BEEN SHOWN TO HAVE A POOR AFFECT ON SLEEP. TRY READING, FOCUSING ON YOUR BREATH, GUIDED MEDITATIONS, YOGA NIDRA, OR MUSCLE TENSE BREATH IN APPENDIX B TO HELP YOU DRIFT OFF TO DREAMLAND AT AN EARLY HOUR TO GET IN A GOOD NIGHT'S REST.

CHAPTER 10
MINDFUL MOVEMENT

"LACK OF TIME IS ACTUALLY LACK OF PRIORITIES"
–TIM FERRISS

MOVEMENT GETS YOU INTO YOUR BODY AND OUT OF THE WORRIES, ANGER, SADNESS, ETC IN YOUR HEAD. MINDFUL MOVEMENT IS FOCUSING ON WHAT YOUR PHYSICAL BODY IS DOING INSTEAD OF BEING CAUGHT IN THE TORNADO OF THOUGHTS WE USUALLY LET RUN THE SHOW. BEING MINDFUL DURING MOVEMENT MEANS BRINGING ATTENTION AND AWARENESS TO YOUR BODY. YOUR ARMS, LEGS, TORSO, ETC. HOW IT IS MOVING, HOW DOES IT FEEL, AND WHAT SENSATIONS ARE YOU EXPERIENCING? ALSO NOTICING YOUR THOUGHTS AND FEELINGS RELATED TO THE MOVEMENT YOU HAVE CHOSEN. ARE YOUR THOUGHTS NEGATIVE OR POSITIVE? IS IT TRYING TO CONVINCE YOU THAT THIS IS BS OR TO STOP ALTOGETHER? RECOGNIZING ALL THESE THINGS IS VERY HELPFUL IN A MINDFUL WEIGHT LOSS JOURNEY.

WE CAN'T IGNORE THE NUMEROUS BENEFITS OF EXERCISE. MENTAL, PHYSICAL, EVEN EMOTIONAL. INSTANT BENEFITS AND LONG TERM BUT IF YOU ARE ANYTHING LIKE ME, YOUR RELATIONSHIP WITH EXERCISE ISN'T GREAT. IT'S PROBABLY ALL OR NOTHING. SIX INTENSE WORKOUTS A WEEK OR NOT AT ALL. IT'S FORCED, NOT ENJOYED, AND YOU'RE FIGHTING IT THE WHOLE WAY.

CHANGING THE WAY YOU VIEW PHYSICAL ACTIVITY CAN BE THE BEST THING FOR BODY TRANSFORMATION. BY ALTERING THIS MINDSET, YOU BEGIN TO WANT TO DO IT AND ENJOY IT. DON'T GET ME WRONG, SOME DAYS I DON'T HAVE A HUGE DESIRE TO MOVE AND HAVE TO PUSH MYSELF. I DO IT BECAUSE I KNOW IT FEELS GOOD AFTER. THE SENSE OF ACCOMPLISHMENT, THE MOTIVATION, AND ENERGY GAINED MEANS I NEVER REGRET PUSHING MYSELF TO GET IT DONE.

IT'S IMPORTANT TO CHANGE THE WAY YOU VIEW EXERCISE. FOR ME, IT USED TO BE SOMETHING I DID IN ORDER TO MAKE MY BODY SMALLER AND I IGNORED ALL THE OTHER PROFOUND BENEFITS. IF I WASN'T ACTIVELY DIETING, THEN I WASN'T EXERCISING EITHER. THE ALL OR NOTHING PLAN AFFECTED EVERY ASPECT.

I BEGAN TO CHANGE MY MINDSET AROUND PHYSICAL ACTIVITY. IT BECAME SOMETHING THAT WAS FOR ME. I WANTED TO SEE WHAT MY BODY COULD DO AND CHANGING IT IN THE PROCESS WAS JUST A PERK. I FOUND THINGS I LIKED TO DO. LIFTING WEIGHTS AND YOGA. WEIGHTS MADE ME FEEL STRONG AND CONFIDENT. WHILE YOGA CONNECTED ME TO MY BODY IN A WAY I HAVE NEVER EXPERIENCED. MAYBE YOU'LL LIKE YOGA, PILATES, DANCE, HIIT, OR CYCLING. TRY DIFFERENT THINGS AND FIND SOMETHING THAT FITS YOU. WAIT UNTIL THE END OF THE WORKOUT TO DETERMINE IF YOU'D DO IT AGAIN. CHECK IN WITH YOURSELF AFTER. HOW ARE YOU FEELING? A LITTLE FATIGUED BUT OTHERWISE GOOD AND GAINED A SENSE OF ACHIEVEMENT? THEN STICK WITH THAT AND ADD IN OTHER THINGS AS YOU SEE FIT. TRUST YOURSELF TO FIND AND KNOW WHAT'S MEANT FOR YOU. FITNESS IS NOT ONE SIZE FITS ALL.

I ALSO CHANGED MY WORDING AROUND EXERCISE. I BEGAN CALLING IT MOVEMENT. HUMANS WERE MADE TO MOVE, NOT JUST NETFLIX AND CHILL. CALLING IT MOVEMENT MADE IT SOUND LIKE I WAS DOING SOMETHING POSITIVE FOR MYSELF, NOT THE TORTUOUS BODY HATING WORKOUT JUST SO I COULD JUSTIFY HAVING A PIECE OF CAKE. MOVEMENT IS SELF CARE.
I ASK MYSELF EVERY DAY "WHAT MOVEMENT AM I GETTING IN TODAY?".

NOW THAT I HAVE A NATURAL RELATIONSHIP WITH ACTIVITY, EACH DAY CAN LOOK DIFFERENT. SOME DAYS I CHOOSE CALM, RESTORATIVE EXERCISE LIKE WALKING OR YOGA. OTHER DAYS, I EXPEND ENERGY LIFTING WEIGHTS. I JUST MAKE SURE TO GET MY MOVEMENT IN. IF YOUR DAY IS USUALLY FULL OF WORK AND FAMILY, TRY GETTING UP BEFORE THEY RISE. THIS WILL GIVE YOU SOME TIME TO YOURSELF TO BE IN YOUR BODY WHILE MOVING IT. GETTING UP EARLY CAN BE A HARD HABIT TO BEGIN SO START WITH RISING 15 MINUTES EARLIER THAN NORMAL. THAT'S TOTALLY DOABLE! BUILD ON THAT TIME EACH WEEK TO WHERE YOU ARE GETTING UP EARLY ENOUGH TO GET IN A 30-60 MINUTE WORKOUT.

SOMETIMES IF WE ARE FEELING DOWN AND SLUGGISH, WE JUST NEED TO MOVE OUR BODY. GET BLOOD PUMPING AND HEART RATE UP TO FEEL AN INCREASE IN ENERGY. THE RELEASE OF FEEL GOOD HORMONES THAT YOU GET FROM BEING ACTIVE MEANS YOU WILL NEVER BE DISAPPOINTED THAT YOU CHOSE TO GET IN YOUR DAILY MOVEMENT. THERE IS A SENSE OF ACCOMPLISHMENT AS WELL AT THE END OF A WORKOUT WHEN YOU PROVE TO YOURSELF YOU CAN DO HARD THINGS. IT'S ONLY 30-60 MINUTES OF YOUR DAY. YOU STILL HAVE PLENTY OF TIME FOR OTHER TASKS! ALL THESE PERKS PROVE YOU NEED TO BE MOVING. SOME DAYS YOU WILL LACK THE MOTIVATION TO GET GOING, CHECK OUT THE BOOK THE 5 SECOND RULE BY MEL ROBBINS. YOU CAN 5-4-3-2-1 YOUR WAY TO YOUR WORKOUT.

IF YOU DON'T KNOW WHERE TO START IN FINDING AN ACTIVITY THAT YOU LIKE, YOUTUBE IS FULL OF FREE FITNESS VIDEOS YOU CAN DO FROM THE COMFORT OF YOUR LIVING ROOM. BE SPECIFIC WHEN SEARCHING. INCLUDE THE TIME YOU ARE WANTING THE VIDEO TO LAST, EX: 15 MIN, 30 MIN, 45 MIN. PLUS THE BODY AREA YOU WANT TO WORK, EX: LEGS, ABS, FULL BODY, ETC. DON'T FORGET TO ADD IN SPECIFICS LIKE LOW IMPACT, STRENGTH TRAINING, OR BODY WEIGHT TO GET THE EXACT WORKOUTS YOU WANT TO DO. ONCE THEY COME UP, DON'T OVERTHINK IT AND SCROLL FOR TOO LONG WASTING EXERCISE TIME. GO WITH YOUR GUT OR THE FIRST ONE THAT INTERESTS YOU, PICK AND START! AN EVEN BETTER THING TO DO IS PICK THE VIDEO THE NIGHT BEFORE, SO YOU KNOW THE PLAN FOR THE NEXT MORNING.

THINK BACK TO YOUR "WHY" FROM THE PREVIOUS JOURNAL PAGES. THAT STATEMENT WILL HELP YOU TO FOCUS ON A REASON FOR MOVEMENT THAT IS NOT ONLY A PHYSICAL GOAL. YES, WEIGHT LOSS IS A PERK OF WORKING OUT AND HAVING AN ACTIVE LIFESTYLE BUT WHAT'S A DEEPER REASON? SO YOU CAN PLAY WITH YOUR KIDS OR GRANDKIDS WITHOUT GETTING WINDED? BEING ABLE TO CARRY ALL YOUR GROCERIES IN AT ONE TIME? CARRYING TWO KIDS AT ONE TIME? HAVING BETTER MOVEMENT TO GET UP FROM A CHAIR OR OUT OF THE BATHTUB? THERE ARE MANY WAYS THAT YOUR LIFE CAN IMPROVE BY MAKING THE CHOICE TO MOVE YOUR BODY CONSISTENTLY. YOU JUST HAVE TO LOOK FOR THEM. MAKE THEM YOUR MOTIVATION TO GET UP WHEN STAYING ON THE COUCH SOUNDS BETTER THAN MOVING YOUR BODY. THE COUCH WILL ALWAYS BE THERE. TAKE THE TIME TO CHOOSE TO BETTER YOUR BODY, NURTURE IT, AND SEE WHAT IT CAN DO.

CONCLUSION

THE ACTIVITIES, PROMPTS, AND HABITS IN THIS BOOK BRING SELF AWARENESS. BEING AWARE OF WHY YOU DO WHAT YOU DO BRINGS CLARITY AND THE ABILITY TO THEN CHANGE IN ANY WAY THAT YOU DESIRE. IT COULD BE BECAUSE OF A HABIT, A BELIEF, OR A VOICE IN YOUR HEAD. AS SOON AS YOU BRING YOUR AWARENESS TO THOSE THINGS YOU ARE INSTANTLY MORE APT TO CREATE TRANSFORMATION. THE REAL WORK COMES IN NOTICING WHEN IT'S A HABIT, BELIEF, OR VOICE IN YOUR HEAD THAT'S CREATING THE REALITY YOU DON'T DESIRE. IT'S LIKE THE LAYERS OF AN ONION. EVERY LAYER YOU LEARN SOMETHING NEW AND HOW TO REFRAME IT TO BENEFIT YOUR SUCCESS!

IN THIS LEARNING PROCESS ALLOW YOURSELF TO BE A STUDENT. YOU'RE LEARNING A NEW WAY OF EATING AND BEING WITH FOOD. AND ALSO HOW TO CALL YOURSELF OUT ON YOUR OWN BS. THE LEARNING EXPERIENCES WILL COME WHEN YOU HAVE A BROWNIE MID DAY BUT YOU AREN'T HUNGRY OR YOU OVEREAT WHILE OUT WITH FRIENDS. GIVE YOURSELF SOME GRACE IN THESE MOMENTS, KNOWING THAT YOU ARE TRANSFORMING FOREVER. THIS WAY OF LIVING IS A MARATHON, NOT A SHORTCUT OR A SPRINT. YOU WILL LEARN THAT YOU CAN TRUST YOUR BODY TO HANDLE WHAT YOU TAKE IN WITHOUT GAINING WEIGHT BECAUSE YOU LISTEN WHEN IT'S FULL AND WAIT TO EAT AGAIN UNTIL YOU ARE TRULY HUNGRY. AND IF FOR SOME REASON YOU DON'T QUITE STICK TO A HABIT FOR ONE MEAL, THERE IS ALWAYS THE NEXT MEAL TO GO BACK TO HABIT PRACTICE AND LISTENING TO YOUR BODY.

OF UTMOST IMPORTANCE... CHANGE IS NOT A STRAIGHT LINE. YOU WILL HAVE UPS AND DOWNS, GOODS AND BADS. THEY ARE ALL LEARNING EXPERIENCES THAT TEACH YOU WHAT WORKS AND WHAT DOESN'T. LEARN FROM THE EXPERIENCES AND RETURN TO YOUR HABITS.

LEARN AND RETURN!!

AND FINAL THOUGHT... LET GO OF THE TIMELINE! THIS IS FOR THE REST OF YOUR LIFE. TO TRULY CHANGE THE WAY YOU INTERACT WITH FOOD, NOT JUST LOSE WEIGHT FOR A WEDDING OR VACATION. THERE IS NO GOAL POST OF LOSE X POUNDS BY THIS DATE. THIS IS HOW YOU LOSE WEIGHT AND KEEP IT OFF. YOU NEVER GO ON OR OFF AGAIN, YOU JUST LEARN AND RETURN.

CHEERS TO CHANGE!

IF YOU FOUND THIS JOURNAL HELPFUL, SHARE WITH FRIENDS AND FAMILY OR LEAVE A LOVELY REVIEW ON AMAZON. THIS WILL MAKE IT EASIER FOR OTHERS TO FIND SO THEY CAN GET STARTED ON THEIR JOURNEY TO FOOD FREEDOM AND BODY CHANGE.

APPENDIX A
POSITIVE BODY IMAGE

MINDFULNESS APPLIES TO ALL AREAS OF LIFE, INCLUDING BODY IMAGE. BEING MINDFUL WHEN IT COMES TO THE IMAGE YOU HAVE OF YOURSELF BRINGS TO AWARENESS PATTERNS, THOUGHTS, AND FEELINGS. IF YOU REFLECT BACK TO THE "NAME THE PLAYERS" JOURNAL SHEET, DID YOU HAVE A PLAYER FOR BODY IMAGE? BODY IMAGE BETTY WAS THE CHARACTER IN MY HEAD ALWAYS MAKING NEGATIVE JUDGEMENTS ABOUT MY BODY. SIMPY BEING MINDFUL AND AWARE OF BETTY'S EXISTENCE GAVE ME THE ABILITY TO NOT IDENTIFY WITH HER AND SLOWLY INCREASE MY SELF CONFIDENCE.

WHEN WE ARE OUT OF TOUCH WITH OUR BODY'S AND MINDFULNESS, THERE TENDS TO BE A TYPICAL CYCLE OF DESIRE TO CHANGE YOUR BODY. IT STARTS WITH 1) WEIGHT GAIN, 2) FEEL BAD ABOUT IT, 3) TRY TO LOSE IT, 4) USE FOOD AS COMFORT WHEN LIFE IS HARD AND DIETING SUCKS, 5) GAIN MORE WEIGHT, 6) FEEL WORSE, AND 7) DEVELOP THE "IT'S HOPELESS AND NOTHING WORKS FOR ME" MENTALITY. IN ORDER TO STOP THE NEGATIVE CYCLE, WORKING TO IMPROVE BODY IMAGE AND HABITS GETS YOU IN TUNE WITH YOUR BODY SO IT CAN ALL WORK TOGETHER! WHEN WE IMPROVE THE WAY WE SEE OUR BODY WE STOP THE "FEEL BAD" WHICH MEANS YOU DON'T TURN TO FOOD FOR COMFORT, YOU DON'T GAIN MORE WEIGHT, AND THE CYCLE ENDS!

BY ACCEPTING OUR BODY AND APPRECIATING ALL IT DOES FOR US, WE CAN MOVE FORWARD INTO NEUTRALITY OR POSITIVITY RELATED TO OUR PHYSICALNESS WHICH HELPS TO END THE DIETING AND FOOD OBSESSION. WE DEVELOP AN ACCEPTANCE OR "IT IS, WHAT IT IS" ATTITUDE ABOUT OUR BODY AS WE TAKE POSITIVE ACTION TO IMPROVE THE HEALTH AND MOBILITY OF IT.

CONSIDER EVERYTHING YOUR BODY ALLOWS YOU TO DO! WALK, DANCE, HUG, HAVE SEX, RUN, BE HERE ON EARTH, ETC. LITERALLY YOU WOULD NOT BE PRESENT ON THIS EARTH WITHOUT IT. STOP AND THINK ABOUT ALL THE THINGS IT DOES WITHOUT BEING ASKED. LUNGS BREATHING, HEART BEATING, FOOD DIGESTING, HORMONES SECRETING, AND MUSCLES MOVING. ALL ON ITS OWN WITHOUT AWARENESS OR EFFORTS FROM YOU. ALL OF THIS PROVES THAT YOUR BODY IS MAGICAL AND IT'S WORTHY OF APPRECIATION.

COMPASSION AND FORGIVENESS FOR YOUR BODY CAN GO A LONG WAY TO HEALING YOUR RELATIONSHIP WITH IT AND MOVING YOU ALONG THE PATH TO SELF TRUST AND SELF CONFIDENCE. YOUR BODY MAY NOT HAVE ALWAYS DONE WHAT YOU WANTED IT TO. IT MAY NOT HAVE BEEN THE EXACT WAY THAT OUR SOCIETY SAYS IT NEEDS TO BE IN ORDER FOR IT TO BE CONSIDERED A "GOOD" BODY. THAT DOESN'T MEAN THAT WE CAN'T BE THANKFUL FOR WHAT IT IS CAPABLE OF. OR HAVE COMPASSION PLUS LOVE FOR IT WHILE YOU ARE CHANGING YOUR HABITS IN ORDER TO MAKE IT THE BEST VERSION IT CAN BE.

TO START, FORGIVE YOUR BODY FOR THE WAYS YOU FEEL LIKE IT HAS FAILED YOU. MAYBE IT'S RELATED TO HEALTH, FERTILITY, WEIGHT GAIN, NOT ENOUGHNESS, OR A MILLION OTHER REASONS WE NEGATIVELY JUDGE OUR BODIES. PUT YOUR HANDS ON YOUR HEART AND SAY OUT LOUD (OR IN YOUR HEAD) "I FORGIVE YOU" OR "I LOVE YOU" OR "I AM LEARNING TO TRUST YOU".
DO THIS PRACTICE ANYTIME YOU HAVE A NEGATIVE BODY THOUGHT. THIS PRACTICE RELEASES THE NEGATIVITY AROUND YOUR SHAPE AND ALLOWS SPACE FOR SOMETHING POSITIVE TO TAKE ITS PLACE. THE CONSISTENT USE OF THIS PRACTICE WILL DRASTICALLY CHANGE YOUR PERCEPTION OF YOUR BODY.

POSITIVE BODY IMAGE STARTS FROM THE INSIDE. SAYING NICE THINGS TO YOUR BODY IN THE MIRROR NOW IS HOW YOU CAN MAKE BIG CHANGES ON THE OUTSIDE IN THE COMING WEEKS. THE INSIDE REFLECTS THE OUTSIDE! WE TEND TO THINK THAT PINCHING, POKING, PULLING, PRODDING, MAKING NEGATIVE COMMENTS, AND HATING IT TO THE MAX WILL MAKE IT CONFORM TO SOCIETY'S VERSION OF "GOOD". THIS DOESN'T WORK! CHOOSE TO LOVE IT THE WAY IT IS NOW! CHOOSE TO BE GRATEFUL NOW SO YOU CAN BE IN A POSITIVE MINDSET TO TAKE ACTION IN CREATING THE NEWER, BETTER VERSION. INSTEAD OF NEGATIVE COMMENTS ABOUT YOUR FRAME, PRACTICE SAYING NICE OR NEUTRAL THINGS. FOCUS ON SOMETHING LIKABLE OR TOLERABLE ABOUT YOUR BODY RATHER THAN THE CONSTANT NEGATIVE. BY DOING THIS, EVENTUALLY THE NEGATIVITY GETS QUIETER AND NEUTRALITY OR POSITIVITY MOVES IN.

I REALIZE THIS IS VERY COUNTERINTUITIVE FOR OUR SOCIETY. WE HAVE BEEN TAUGHT WE CAN'T LOVE OUR BODIES UNTIL IT'S SKINNY, LEAN, OR TONED. BUT I PROMISE YOUR BODY IS WORTHY OF LOVE NOW! CHECK OUT THE BOOK "BODY POSITIVE POWER" BY MEGAN JAYNE CRABBE.

A GOOD POINT TO MAKE TO THOSE OF US THAT HAVE BEEN SUCCESSFUL IN DIETING AND RESTRICTING TO LOSE WEIGHT... WERE YOU EVER ACTUALLY ANY HAPPIER AT A SMALLER NUMBER/SIZE? OR DID YOU THINK YOU ALWAYS NEEDED TO LOSE MORE OR IT WAS NEVER GOOD ENOUGH? THE OUTSIDE IS NEVER GOOD ENOUGH BECAUSE WE DIDN'T DO THE INNER WORK. WE ALWAYS THOUGHT WE NEEDED TO BE SMALLER, THINNER, MORE TONED, ETC.

KEY TAKEAWAY... MINDSET AND INNER WORK ARE JUST AS IMPORTANT AS OUTER WORK! THE BODY LISTENS TO THE MIND. READ THAT AGAIN. THE BODY LISTENS TO THE MIND!! APPRECIATION OF IT LEADS TO MEETING GOALS. SHAME AND LOATHING LEADS TO MORE GUILT AND NOT ENOUGHNESS. PUT IN WHAT YOU WANT TO GET OUT.

POSITIVE BODY IMAGE ACTIONS AND EXERCISES

IN THE FOLLOWING PAGES, YOU WILL FIND JOURNALING AND ACTIVITIES. THESE WILL HELP YOU TO CREATE AN IMPROVED IMAGE OF SELF. MY GOAL IS THAT YOU SEE HOW WONDERFUL YOUR BODY TRULY IS AND HOW MUCH IT DOES FOR YOU. THESE PAGES AND PRACTICES WILL BEGIN TO TRANSFORM YOUR RELATIONSHIP WITH YOUR EXTERIOR.

A SUPER SIMPLE METHOD FOR SELF LOVE... LOOK INTO YOUR OWN EYES IN THE MIRROR AND SAY "I LOVE YOU" TO YOURSELF 5-10 TIMES. DO THIS WHILE BRUSHING YOUR TEETH. THIS IS CALLED HABIT STACKING. COMPLETING A NEW ACTION (EYE GAZING PLUS "I LOVE YOU") WITH A HABIT YOU ALREADY COMPLETE (BRUSHING TEETH) IS A SOLID WAY TO ADD IN SOMETHING NEW AND INSURE THAT IT GETS DONE!

ACTIVITY 1- CANDLE LIT MIRROR ACTIVITY- LIGHT A CANDLE IN THE BATHROOM NEAR A MIRROR. STANDING IN THE SOFT GLOWING LIGHT OF THE CANDLE, ADMIRE AND CARESS YOUR BODY. START WITH AN AREA YOU FEEL MOST COMFORTABLE WITH, SLOWLY CONTINUE TO OTHER AREAS, AND EVENTUALLY ADMIRE YOUR BODY AS A WHOLE. AS NEGATIVE THOUGHTS ARISE, SEE THEM WITH COMPASSION. WE HAVE BEEN TRAINED TO THINK WE ARE UNLOVEABLE THE WAY WE ARE. REPLACE THE NEGATIVE THOUGHT WITH A POSITIVE OR NEUTRAL STATEMENT, THINKING BACK TO THE LIST OF WONDERFUL THINGS YOUR BODY DOES. ON THE FOLLOWING JOURNAL PAGE, WRITE DOWN YOUR REACTION TO THIS ACTIVITY. DO THIS EXERCISE MANY TIMES AND WRITE YOUR FEEDBACK ON A SEPARATE PIECE OF PAPER. THIS WILL ALLOW YOU TO LOOK BACK LATER AND SEE HOW FAR YOU'VE COME!

ACTIVITY 2- DEAR BODY LETTER- INSTRUCTIONS ON THE PAGE. RETURN TO THIS LETTER WHEN YOU NEED A PICK ME UP RELATED TO BODY IMAGE.

CANDLE LIGHT MIRROR ACTIVITY JOURNAL PAGE

DATE

FREE WRITE: LIST YOUR REACTIONS BELOW, YOUR EMOTIONS, FEELINGS, THOUGHTS, ANYTHING THAT CAME UP

_____

_____

_____

_____

_____

_____

_____

_____

_____

_____

_____

_____

BECAUSE MIRROR WORK CAN BE TRIGGERING AND UPSETTING FOR SOME, BE SURE TO LIST SOME NEUTRAL OR POSITIVE THINGS ABOUT YOUR BODY IN THIS SECTION

_____

_____

_____

_____

_____

DEAR BODY LETTER

DATE

WRITING A LETTER TO YOUR BODY GIVES YOU THE OPPORTUNITY TO THANK IT FOR
ALL THAT IT DOES! AS YOU BRING ATTENTION TO THEM, YOU WILL BE AMAZED AT ALL
THE THINGS YOU TAKE FOR GRANTED! IT DOES SO MUCH! IT'S TIME TO SHOW IT SOME
APPRECIATION. I LIKE TO START AT MY HEAD AND MOVE DOWN. MY EYES ALLOW ME
TO SEE, MY MOUTH SMILES AT OTHERS, MY NOSE ALLOWS ME TO SMELL AMAZING
SCENTS, MY HEART BEATS AND LUNGS BREATHE ON THEIR OWN! MY ARMS HUG,
ABDOMEN DIGESTS FOOD OR MAKES MORE HUMANS! MY LEGS MOVE ME AROUND
AND MY BUM GIVES MY HUSBAND SOMETHING TO SQUEEZE. LIST ALLLL THE THINGS!
REVEL IN THANKS FOR THE VESSEL THAT ALLOWS YOU TO BE HERE ON EARTH!

DEAR BODY:

_____

_____

_____

_____

_____

_____

_____

_____

_____

_____

_____

_____

SINCERELY YOURS,

_____

PS: I PROMISE TO NO LONGER TAKE YOU FOR GRANTED! I SEE ALL YOU DO!

APPENDIX B
RELAXATION AND FOCUS TECHNIQUES

THIS SECTION HAS YOUR GO-TO TECHNIQUES FOR RELAXING, LETTING GO, AND BEING IN THE PRESENT MOMENT. THESE ARE SIMPLE MINDFULNESS TOOLS THAT YOU CAN USE ANYWHERE AND ANYTIME. TRY THEM ALL AND REUSE THE ONES THAT YOU PREFER.

FOCUS ON YOUR BREATH

BREATHING IS SOMETHING WE TEND TO NOT NOTICE BECAUSE IT'S INVOLUNTARILY DONE BY OUR BODY AND NOT SOMETHING WE HAVE TO WORRY ABOUT. WHICH IS GREAT BECAUSE IF WE HAD TO THINK ABOUT BREATHING WE PROBABLY WOULDN'T LAST VERY LONG. BUT IF YOU THINK ABOUT IT, AT ITS CORE, AIR/BREATH IS LIFE. WE CAN DO WITHOUT WATER FOR DAYS AND WITHOUT FOOD FOR WEEKS. BUT WITHOUT AIR... IN MINUTES THE AVERAGE PERSON WOULD DIE. SO TAKING SOME TIME TO BRING YOUR ATTENTION TO THIS LIFE GIVING ESSENCE CAN DECREASE STRESS AND BRING PEACE.

TO BEGIN, SIMPLY CLOSE YOUR EYES AND SET THE INTENTION TO BE AWARE OF YOUR BREATH. AS YOU INHALE DEEPLY THROUGH YOUR NOSE, FOCUS ON FILLING YOUR BELLY WITH AIR LIKE A BALLOON. MOST OF US TEND TO BREATHE INTO THE CHEST. CHEST BREATHING DOESN'T ALLOW FOR THE DEEPER BREATHS THAT BELLY BREATHING CAN, SO PAYING ATTENTION TO WHERE YOU ARE BREATHING IS IMPORTANT. AS YOU EXHALE OUT OF THE MOUTH, FOCUS ON PULLING YOUR BELLY IN AND TOWARDS YOUR SPINE TO SQUEEZE ALL THE AIR BACK OUT.

REPEAT IN THROUGH YOUR NOSE AND OUT THROUGH YOUR MOUTH FOR SEVERAL ROUNDS. FOLLOW YOUR BREATH FROM YOUR NOSE INTO YOUR BELLY AND BACK OUT THROUGH YOUR MOUTH.

OTHER THINGS TO NOTICE AS YOU BREATHE- WHAT DOES IT FEEL AND SOUND LIKE AS IT ENTERS YOUR NOSE? WHAT SENSATIONS AND DIFFERENCES DO YOU SENSE AS IT EXITS THE LIPS?

IF YOUR MIND STARTS TO WANDER, BRING YOUR AWARENESS BACK TO FILLING THE BELLY WITH AIR AND THE SENSATIONS INVOLVED WITH THIS ACTIVITY.

I SUGGEST SETTING A TIMER FOR A SHORT PERIOD OF TIME AND DOING THIS UNTIL IT GOES OFF. OTHERWISE YOU WILL BE CHECKING FREQUENTLY TO SEE HOW LONG YOU'VE BEEN AT IT. YOU CAN START WITH SHORT BURSTS LIKE 3-5 MINUTES AND INCREASE FROM THERE AS YOU GET COMFORTABLE BEING STILL WITH YOUR BREATH.

THE ONLY TECHNIQUE

FOR THIS PRACTICE, YOU WILL PICK SOMETHING TO FOCUS ON. IT CAN BE SOMETHING PRETTY OUTSIDE IN NATURE LIKE A FLOWER OR A TREE. IF YOU DON'T HAVE THE ABILITY TO GO OUTDOORS, IT CAN BE AS SIMPLE AS THE PENCIL HOLDER ON YOUR DESK OR THE STEERING WHEEL OF YOUR CAR.

ONCE YOU HAVE PICKED THE ITEM YOU WILL FOCUS ON, SET A TIMER FOR A MINIMUM OF 3-5 MINUTES. AFTER SETTING THE TIMER TAKE A FEW DEEP BREATHS TO CENTER AND BRING YOURSELF INTO THE PRESENT MOMENT. WHEN THE ITEM HAS YOUR FULL ATTENTION AND AWARENESS, BEGIN TO TAKE IN ALL THE DETAILS OF IT.

YOU ARE ESSENTIALLY PRETENDING TO BE AN ALIEN THAT HAS NEVER SEEN THIS THING AND YOU WANT TO NOTICE EVERY FEATURE IT HAS! USE YOUR 5 SENSES (SEE, TOUCH, SMELL, HEAR, AND TASTE) TO REALLY CONSIDER EVERY ASPECT. LOOK FOR CHARACTERISTICS YOU'VE NEVER PAID ATTENTION TO. CONTINUE DOING THIS FOCUSING TECHNIQUE UNTIL THE TIMER GOES OFF. AFTER A FEW ATTEMPTS AT THIS, FEEL FREE TO EXTEND THE TIME IN ORDER TO FLEX THAT MINDFULNESS MUSCLE.

UNDOUBTEDLY WHEN YOU ARE TRYING TO FOCUS, DISTRACTING THOUGHTS MAY COME IN TO SUGGEST THAT YOU PICK UP DINNER, LET THE DOG OUT, OR DROP JOHNNY OFF AT PRACTICE. THANK THE THOUGHT FOR THE REMINDER AND SWEEP IT AWAY. TELLING YOURSELF THAT THE ONLY THING IN YOUR AWARENESS RIGHT NOW IS THIS ITEM YOU HAVE PICKED TO FOCUS ON. SAYING TO YOURSELF "ONLY ___, ONLY ___, ONLY ___". BRINGING YOUR FOCUS SOLELY BACK TO THIS ITEM "YOU'VE NEVER SEEN BEFORE."

AT THE END WHEN THE TIMER GOES OFF, THANK THE ITEM FOR IT'S PRESENCE AND BEAUTIFUL DETAILS. MORE IMPORTANTLY, THANK YOURSELF FOR TAKING THE TIME TO GET OUT OF YOUR HEAD AND WORK ON BEING MINDFUL TODAY.

WHAT DO YOU SENSE?

WE'VE TALKED SEVERAL TIMES ABOUT USING THE 5 SENSES TO BRING YOURSELF INTO THE PRESENT MOMENT. TRY IT ANYWHERE WITH ANYTHING TO CENTER AND GROUND YOURSELF. YOU CAN EVEN PRACTICE WITH YOUR KIDS. IF THEY ARE FAMILIAR WITH THEM, ASK THEM TO PICK ONE OF THE 5 SENSES THEN USE IT IN THE CURRENT ENVIRONMENT. FOR KIDDOS THAT AREN'T FULLY AWARE OF THEIR 5 SENSES, SIMPLY ASK THEM WHAT THEY HEAR, SEE, FEEL, TASTE, OR SMELL.

MUSCLE TENSION BREATH

WE TEND TO CARRY TENSION IN OUR FACES (EYES, FOREHEAD, MOUTH), SHOULDERS, AND OTHER BODY PARTS. UNCONSCIOUSLY HOLDING TENSION IN THESE AREAS MAKES IT HARD TO BE AT PEACE. THIS METHOD HELPS TO RELEASE TENSION FROM THESE AREAS AND INVOKE STRESS RELIEF.

START BY TAKING A DEEP BREATH IN. FOCUS ON FILLING YOUR BELLY WITH AIR. AFTER YOUR DEEP BREATH IN (WHILE HOLDING THE BREATH) YOU WILL SQUEEZE EVERY MUSCLE FROM TOES TO HEAD. I BEGIN SQUEEZING AT MY FEET, MOVE UP TO CALVES, THIGHS, BUM, CORE, SHOULDERS, ARMS, FISTS, AND LASTLY FACE. HOLD THIS MUSCLE TENSION ALONG WITH YOUR BREATH FOR 5 SECONDS. WHEN THE COUNT OF 5 IS UP, RELAX YOUR BODY AND LET OUT A BIG SIGHING EXHALE WITH AN AHHHH SOUND.

REPEAT THIS AT LEAST 3-5 TIMES OR AS MANY TIMES AS NEEDED UNTIL YOU FEEL MORE CONTENT, PRESENT, AND RELAXED IN YOUR BODY.

BREATH COUNTING

COUNTING YOUR BREATH IS AN EASY WAY TO STAY FOCUSED AND MINDFUL OF YOUR BREATHING. NUMBERING YOUR INHALES, EXHALES, AND HOLDS KEEPS YOUR MIND ATTENTIVE AND LESS LIKELY TO WANDER. YOU WILL COUNT IN YOUR HEAD OR ON YOUR FINGERS.

BREATH COUNTING IN ITS SIMPLEST FORM IS TO:
(1) INHALE WHILE YOU COUNT TO 4,
(2) HOLD WHILE YOU COUNT TO 4,
(3) EXHALE WHILE YOU COUNT TO 4, AND
(4) HOLD WHILE YOU COUNT TO 4.

THEN START OVER. INHALE FOR 4, HOLD FOR 4, EXHALE FOR 4, AND HOLD FOR 4 AGAIN. REPEAT THE CYCLE 5-10 TIMES OR UNTIL YOU FEEL MORE CALM.

YOU CAN ALTER THIS WAY OF BREATHING TO SUIT YOURSELF. IF YOU CAN'T HOLD FOR 4, THEN SHORTEN IT. THE IMPORTANT THING IS TO BRING YOUR AWARENESS TO COUNTING AND BREATHING INSTEAD OF ANYTHING IN THE EXTERNAL ENVIRONMENT.

IF YOU'VE MASTERED THE EQUAL COUNTS OF 4 TO INHALE, EXHALE, AND HOLD, AN ALTERNATE WAY TO BREATH COUNT IS EXTENDING THE EXHALE TO BE LONGER THAN THE INHALE. FOR EXAMPLE, WHEN INHALING FOR 4, TRY EXHALING FOR A COUNT OF 6. YOU CAN ALSO EXTEND THE INHALE TO 6 AND EXHALE TO A COUNT OF 8. FEEL FREE TO HOLD FOR ANY COUNT THAT YOU LIKE. PLAY AROUND WITH WHAT METHOD FEELS GOOD FOR YOU AND KEEP PRACTICING!

FOCUS ON YOUR FEET

WHEN YOUR THOUGHTS ARE SPIRALING IN FEAR, WORRY, ANGST, IMPATIENCE, OR ANGER, TRY FOCUSING ON THE BODY PART THAT IS FURTHEST FROM YOUR THOUGHTS. YOUR FEET!!

HOW DO THEY FEEL ON THE GROUND? WHAT IS THE TEXTURE OF THE SURFACE BELOW THEM? WHICH PARTS OF YOUR FEET ARE TOUCHING THE GROUND? IS THE WEIGHT EQUALLY DISTRIBUTED? IF YOU MOVE AROUND WHAT DOES IT FEEL LIKE AS YOU PICK THEM UP AND SET THEM BACK DOWN. IF YOU MOVE FROM THE HARD FLOOR TO A RUG/CARPET OR VICE VERSA, NOTICE THE CHANGE. SPREAD, FLEX, CURL, AND EXTEND YOUR TOES, BRINGING FOCUS TO THE SENSATION EACH MOVEMENT BRINGS. PUSH THROUGH YOUR FEET INTO THE GROUND TO BRING FULL AWARENESS TO ONLY THIS BODY PART.

PAYING ATTENTION TO EVERY DETAIL OF THE THINGS THAT CARRY YOU THROUGH LIFE IS A WAY TO GROUND AND CENTER YOURSELF. IT BRINGS YOU INTO YOUR BODY AND OUT OF YOUR THOUGHTS WHICH IS THE BASIS OF MINDFULNESS. YOU CAN VISUALIZE TREE ROOTS GROWING FROM YOUR FEET ANCHORING YOU INTO THE GROUND AND THIS PRESENT MOMENT. EVEN TAKE IT A LITTLE FURTHER BY INVITING GRATITUDE INTO THIS MOMENT TO SHIFT YOUR VIBE. THANK YOUR FEET FOR ALLOWING YOU TO EXPERIENCE LIFE AS THEY BEAR THE WEIGHT OF IT ALL.

APPENDIX C
DAILY, WEEKLY, AND MONTHLY JOURNAL PAGES FOR WEEKS 8-16

DAILY JOURNAL

DATE

TO DO LIST:

_____

_____

_____

TODAY I AM GRATEFUL FOR:

1.

_____

2.

_____

DAILY AFFIRMATION:

_____

CRAVINGS AND MY REACTION TO THEM

_____

_____

_____

_____

WATER TRACKER   ◊◊◊◊◊◊◊

MOVEMENT

_____

MOOD TRACKER   ☹ ☹ ☺ ☺ ☺

HOURS OF SLEEP:

3-4 MEALS, NO SNACKING	YES/NO
HUNGER 30 MINUTES BEFORE BREAKFAST	YES/NO
HUNGER 30 MIN BEFORE LUNCH	YES/NO
HUNGER 30 MIN BEFORE DINNER	YES/NO
AT ALL MEALS, EAT JUST ENOUGH	YES/NO

DAILY FOOD OR BODY WIN

_____

_____

_____

_____

INTENTION SETTING FOR TOMORROW

_____

_____

_____

DAILY JOURNAL

DATE

TO DO LIST:

WATER TRACKER ⬡⬡⬡⬡⬡⬡⬡

MOVEMENT

TODAY I AM GRATEFUL FOR:

MOOD TRACKER ☹ ☹ ☺ ☺ ☺

HOURS OF SLEEP:

1.

3-4 MEALS, NO SNACKING	YES/NO
HUNGER 30 MINUTES BEFORE BREAKFAST	YES/NO
HUNGER 30 MIN BEFORE LUNCH	YES/NO

2.

| HUNGER 30 MIN BEFORE DINNER | YES/NO |
| AT ALL MEALS, EAT JUST ENOUGH | YES/NO |

DAILY AFFIRMATION:

CRAVINGS AND MY REACTION TO THEM

DAILY FOOD OR BODY WIN

INTENTION SETTING FOR TOMORROW

DAILY JOURNAL

DATE

TO DO LIST:

_____

_____

_____

_____

TODAY I AM GRATEFUL FOR:

1. _____

_____

2. _____

_____

DAILY AFFIRMATION:

_____

CRAVINGS AND MY REACTION TO THEM

_____

_____

_____

_____

WATER TRACKER ⬡⬡⬡⬡⬡⬡⬡

MOVEMENT

_____

_____

MOOD TRACKER ☹ ☹ ☺ ☺ ☺

HOURS OF SLEEP:

3-4 MEALS, NO SNACKING   YES/NO

HUNGER 30 MINUTES BEFORE BREAKFAST   YES/NO

HUNGER 30 MIN BEFORE LUNCH   YES/NO

HUNGER 30 MIN BEFORE DINNER   YES/NO

AT ALL MEALS, EAT JUST ENOUGH   YES/NO

DAILY FOOD OR BODY WIN

_____

_____

_____

_____

INTENTION SETTING FOR TOMORROW

_____

_____

_____

DAILY JOURNAL

DATE

TO DO LIST:

WATER TRACKER ◊◊◊◊◊◊◊

MOVEMENT

MOOD TRACKER ☹ ☹ ☺ ☺ ☺

TODAY I AM GRATEFUL FOR:

HOURS OF SLEEP:

1.

3-4 MEALS, NO SNACKING	YES/NO
HUNGER 30 MINUTES BEFORE BREAKFAST	YES/NO
HUNGER 30 MIN BEFORE LUNCH	YES/NO
HUNGER 30 MIN BEFORE DINNER	YES/NO
AT ALL MEALS, EAT JUST ENOUGH	YES/NO

2.

DAILY AFFIRMATION:

CRAVINGS AND MY REACTION TO THEM

DAILY FOOD OR BODY WIN

INTENTION SETTING FOR TOMORROW

DAILY JOURNAL

DATE

TO DO LIST:

_____

_____

_____

TODAY I AM GRATEFUL FOR:

1.

_____

2.

_____

DAILY AFFIRMATION:

_____

CRAVINGS AND MY REACTION TO THEM

_____

_____

_____

_____

WATER TRACKER ○○○○○○○

MOVEMENT

_____

_____

MOOD TRACKER ☹ ☹ ☺ ☺ ☺

HOURS OF SLEEP:

3-4 MEALS, NO SNACKING	YES/NO
HUNGER 30 MINUTES BEFORE BREAKFAST	YES/NO
HUNGER 30 MIN BEFORE LUNCH	YES/NO
HUNGER 30 MIN BEFORE DINNER	YES/NO
AT ALL MEALS, EAT JUST ENOUGH	YES/NO

DAILY FOOD OR BODY WIN

_____

_____

_____

INTENTION SETTING FOR TOMORROW

_____

_____

_____

DAILY JOURNAL

DATE

TO DO LIST:

_____

_____

_____

TODAY I AM GRATEFUL FOR:

1. _____

2. _____

DAILY AFFIRMATION:

_____

CRAVINGS AND MY REACTION TO THEM

_____

_____

_____

_____

INTENTION SETTING FOR TOMORROW

_____

_____

_____

WATER TRACKER ⬡⬡⬡⬡⬡⬡⬡

MOVEMENT

_____

MOOD TRACKER ☹ ☹ ☺ ☺ ☺

HOURS OF SLEEP:

3-4 MEALS, NO SNACKING	YES/NO
HUNGER 30 MINUTES BEFORE BREAKFAST	YES/NO
HUNGER 30 MIN BEFORE LUNCH	YES/NO
HUNGER 30 MIN BEFORE DINNER	YES/NO
AT ALL MEALS, EAT JUST ENOUGH	YES/NO

DAILY FOOD OR BODY WIN

_____

_____

_____

_____

DAILY JOURNAL

DATE

TO DO LIST:

WATER TRACKER ○○○○○○○

MOVEMENT

TODAY I AM GRATEFUL FOR:

MOOD TRACKER 😣 😞 😐 🙂 😊

HOURS OF SLEEP:

1.

3-4 MEALS, NO SNACKING	YES/NO
HUNGER 30 MINUTES BEFORE BREAKFAST	YES/NO
HUNGER 30 MIN BEFORE LUNCH	YES/NO
HUNGER 30 MIN BEFORE DINNER	YES/NO
AT ALL MEALS, EAT JUST ENOUGH	YES/NO

2.

DAILY AFFIRMATION:

CRAVINGS AND MY REACTION TO THEM

DAILY FOOD OR BODY WIN

INTENTION SETTING FOR TOMORROW

WEEKLY JOURNAL

DATE

WEIGHT:

MY WHY...
_____
_____
_____
_____

WHAT IS GOING WELL WITH THIS WEEKS HABIT?
_____
_____
_____
_____

WHAT COULD BE BETTER?
_____
_____
_____
_____

GOALS FOR NEXT WEEK...
_____
_____
_____
_____

MONTHLY JOURNAL

DATE

MEASUREMENTS-

CHEST:

WAIST:

HIPS:

THIGHS: RIGHT-   LEFT-

CALF: RIGHT-   LEFT-

ARMS: RIGHT-   LEFT-

LOOK HOW FAR I'VE COME!!
WRITE DOWN EXAMPLES OF WAYS YOU HAVE IMPROVED IN THE LAST 4 WEEKS

_____

_____

_____

_____

_____

_____

_____

_____

_____

_____

DAILY JOURNAL

DATE

TO DO LIST:

WATER TRACKER ◊◊◊◊◊◊◊

MOVEMENT

MOOD TRACKER 😖 🙁 😐 🙂 😊

TODAY I AM GRATEFUL FOR:

HOURS OF SLEEP:

1.

3-4 MEALS, NO SNACKING	YES/NO
HUNGER 30 MINUTES BEFORE BREAKFAST	YES/NO

2.

HUNGER 30 MIN BEFORE LUNCH	YES/NO
HUNGER 30 MIN BEFORE DINNER	YES/NO

DAILY AFFIRMATION:

AT ALL MEALS, EAT JUST ENOUGH   YES/NO

CRAVINGS AND MY REACTION TO THEM

DAILY FOOD OR BODY WIN

INTENTION SETTING FOR TOMORROW

DAILY JOURNAL

DATE

TO DO LIST:

_____

_____

_____

TODAY I AM GRATEFUL FOR:

1.

2.

DAILY AFFIRMATION:

CRAVINGS AND MY REACTION TO THEM

_____

_____

_____

_____

INTENTION SETTING FOR TOMORROW

_____

_____

_____

WATER TRACKER　◇◇◇◇◇◇◇

MOVEMENT

_____

MOOD TRACKER　☹ ☹ ☺ ☺ ☺

HOURS OF SLEEP:

3-4 MEALS, NO SNACKING　　　　　YES/NO

HUNGER 30 MINUTES BEFORE BREAKFAST　YES/NO

HUNGER 30 MIN BEFORE LUNCH　　　YES/NO

HUNGER 30 MIN BEFORE DINNER　　YES/NO

AT ALL MEALS, EAT JUST ENOUGH　YES/NO

DAILY FOOD OR BODY WIN

_____

_____

_____

_____

DAILY JOURNAL

DATE

TO DO LIST:

_____

_____

_____

TODAY I AM GRATEFUL FOR:

1. _____

_____

2. _____

_____

DAILY AFFIRMATION:

_____

CRAVINGS AND MY REACTION TO THEM

_____

_____

_____

_____

WATER TRACKER ⬡⬡⬡⬡⬡⬡⬡

MOVEMENT

_____

_____

MOOD TRACKER ☹ ☹ ☺ ☺ ☺

HOURS OF SLEEP:

3-4 MEALS, NO SNACKING	YES/NO
HUNGER 30 MINUTES BEFORE BREAKFAST	YES/NO
HUNGER 30 MIN BEFORE LUNCH	YES/NO
HUNGER 30 MIN BEFORE DINNER	YES/NO
AT ALL MEALS, EAT JUST ENOUGH	YES/NO

DAILY FOOD OR BODY WIN

_____

_____

_____

_____

INTENTION SETTING FOR TOMORROW

_____

_____

_____

DAILY JOURNAL

DATE

TO DO LIST:

WATER TRACKER ○○○○○○○

MOVEMENT

TODAY I AM GRATEFUL FOR:

MOOD TRACKER ☹ ☹ ☺ ☺ ☺

HOURS OF SLEEP:

1.

| 3-4 MEALS, NO SNACKING | YES/NO |

2.

| HUNGER 30 MINUTES BEFORE BREAKFAST | YES/NO |

| HUNGER 30 MIN BEFORE LUNCH | YES/NO |

| HUNGER 30 MIN BEFORE DINNER | YES/NO |

DAILY AFFIRMATION:

| AT ALL MEALS, EAT JUST ENOUGH | YES/NO |

CRAVINGS AND MY REACTION TO THEM

DAILY FOOD OR BODY WIN

INTENTION SETTING FOR TOMORROW

DAILY JOURNAL

DATE

TO DO LIST:

WATER TRACKER ⬦⬦⬦⬦⬦⬦⬦

MOVEMENT

TODAY I AM GRATEFUL FOR:

MOOD TRACKER 😣 🙁 😐 🙂 😊

HOURS OF SLEEP:

1.

3-4 MEALS, NO SNACKING	YES/NO

2.

HUNGER 30 MINUTES BEFORE BREAKFAST	YES/NO
HUNGER 30 MIN BEFORE LUNCH	YES/NO

DAILY AFFIRMATION:

HUNGER 30 MIN BEFORE DINNER	YES/NO
AT ALL MEALS, EAT JUST ENOUGH	YES/NO

CRAVINGS AND MY REACTION TO THEM

DAILY FOOD OR BODY WIN

INTENTION SETTING FOR TOMORROW

DAILY JOURNAL

DATE

TO DO LIST:

_____

_____

_____

_____

TODAY I AM GRATEFUL FOR:

1. _____

_____

2. _____

_____

DAILY AFFIRMATION:

_____

CRAVINGS AND MY REACTION TO THEM

_____

_____

_____

_____

_____

WATER TRACKER ◇◇◇◇◇◇◇

MOVEMENT

_____

MOOD TRACKER ☹ ☹ ☺ ☺ ☺

HOURS OF SLEEP:

3-4 MEALS, NO SNACKING	YES/NO
HUNGER 30 MINUTES BEFORE BREAKFAST	YES/NO
HUNGER 30 MIN BEFORE LUNCH	YES/NO
HUNGER 30 MIN BEFORE DINNER	YES/NO
AT ALL MEALS, EAT JUST ENOUGH	YES/NO

DAILY FOOD OR BODY WIN

_____

_____

_____

_____

INTENTION SETTING FOR TOMORROW

_____

_____

_____

DAILY JOURNAL

DATE

TO DO LIST:

WATER TRACKER   ◊◊◊◊◊◊◊

MOVEMENT

MOOD TRACKER   😣 ☹️ 😐 🙂 😊

TODAY I AM GRATEFUL FOR:

HOURS OF SLEEP:

1.

3-4 MEALS, NO SNACKING	YES/NO
HUNGER 30 MINUTES BEFORE BREAKFAST	YES/NO
HUNGER 30 MIN BEFORE LUNCH	YES/NO
HUNGER 30 MIN BEFORE DINNER	YES/NO
AT ALL MEALS, EAT JUST ENOUGH	YES/NO

2.

DAILY AFFIRMATION:

CRAVINGS AND MY REACTION TO THEM

DAILY FOOD OR BODY WIN

INTENTION SETTING FOR TOMORROW

WEEKLY JOURNAL

DATE

WEIGHT:

MY WHY...

_____

_____

_____

_____

WHAT IS GOING WELL WITH THIS WEEKS HABIT?

_____

_____

_____

WHAT COULD BE BETTER?

_____

_____

_____

GOALS FOR NEXT WEEK...

_____

_____

_____

_____

DAILY JOURNAL

DATE

TO DO LIST:

_____

_____

_____

_____

TODAY I AM GRATEFUL FOR:

1. _____

_____

2. _____

_____

DAILY AFFIRMATION:

_____

CRAVINGS AND MY REACTION TO THEM

_____

_____

_____

_____

WATER TRACKER   ○○○○○○○

MOVEMENT

_____

MOOD TRACKER   ☹ ☹ ☺ ☺ ☺

HOURS OF SLEEP:

3-4 MEALS, NO SNACKING	YES/NO
HUNGER 30 MINUTES BEFORE BREAKFAST	YES/NO
HUNGER 30 MIN BEFORE LUNCH	YES/NO
HUNGER 30 MIN BEFORE DINNER	YES/NO
AT ALL MEALS, EAT JUST ENOUGH	YES/NO

DAILY FOOD OR BODY WIN

_____

_____

_____

_____

INTENTION SETTING FOR TOMORROW

_____

_____

_____

DAILY JOURNAL

DATE

TO DO LIST:

WATER TRACKER   ○○○○○○○

MOVEMENT

MOOD TRACKER   😣 😞 😐 🙂 😊

TODAY I AM GRATEFUL FOR:

HOURS OF SLEEP:

1.

3-4 MEALS, NO SNACKING   YES/NO

HUNGER 30 MINUTES BEFORE BREAKFAST   YES/NO

2.

HUNGER 30 MIN BEFORE LUNCH   YES/NO

HUNGER 30 MIN BEFORE DINNER   YES/NO

DAILY AFFIRMATION:

AT ALL MEALS, EAT JUST ENOUGH   YES/NO

CRAVINGS AND MY REACTION TO THEM

DAILY FOOD OR BODY WIN

INTENTION SETTING FOR TOMORROW

DAILY JOURNAL

DATE

TO DO LIST:

WATER TRACKER   ◊ ◊ ◊ ◊ ◊ ◊ ◊

MOVEMENT

MOOD TRACKER   ☹ ☹ 😐 ☺ 😊

TODAY I AM GRATEFUL FOR:

HOURS OF SLEEP:

1.

3-4 MEALS, NO SNACKING	YES/NO
HUNGER 30 MINUTES BEFORE BREAKFAST	YES/NO
HUNGER 30 MIN BEFORE LUNCH	YES/NO
HUNGER 30 MIN BEFORE DINNER	YES/NO
AT ALL MEALS, EAT JUST ENOUGH	YES/NO

2.

DAILY AFFIRMATION:

CRAVINGS AND MY REACTION TO THEM

DAILY FOOD OR BODY WIN

INTENTION SETTING FOR TOMORROW

DAILY JOURNAL

DATE

TO DO LIST:

_____

_____

_____

_____

TODAY I AM GRATEFUL FOR:

1. _____

_____

2. _____

_____

DAILY AFFIRMATION:

_____

CRAVINGS AND MY REACTION TO THEM

_____

_____

_____

_____

_____

WATER TRACKER   ⬭⬭⬭⬭⬭⬭⬭

MOVEMENT

_____

_____

MOOD TRACKER   😣 😟 😐 ☺ 😊

HOURS OF SLEEP:

3-4 MEALS, NO SNACKING	YES/NO
HUNGER 30 MINUTES BEFORE BREAKFAST	YES/NO
HUNGER 30 MIN BEFORE LUNCH	YES/NO
HUNGER 30 MIN BEFORE DINNER	YES/NO
AT ALL MEALS, EAT JUST ENOUGH	YES/NO

DAILY FOOD OR BODY WIN

_____

_____

_____

_____

INTENTION SETTING FOR TOMORROW

_____

_____

_____

DAILY JOURNAL

DATE

TO DO LIST:

WATER TRACKER ⬡⬡⬡⬡⬡⬡⬡

MOVEMENT

TODAY I AM GRATEFUL FOR:

MOOD TRACKER ☹ ☹ ☺ ☺ ☺

HOURS OF SLEEP:

1.

3-4 MEALS, NO SNACKING	YES/NO
HUNGER 30 MINUTES BEFORE BREAKFAST	YES/NO
HUNGER 30 MIN BEFORE LUNCH	YES/NO
HUNGER 30 MIN BEFORE DINNER	YES/NO
AT ALL MEALS, EAT JUST ENOUGH	YES/NO

2.

DAILY AFFIRMATION:

CRAVINGS AND MY REACTION TO THEM

DAILY FOOD OR BODY WIN

INTENTION SETTING FOR TOMORROW

DAILY JOURNAL

DATE

TO DO LIST:

WATER TRACKER ⬠⬠⬠⬠⬠⬠⬠

MOVEMENT

TODAY I AM GRATEFUL FOR:

MOOD TRACKER 😣 😞 😐 🙂 😊

1.

HOURS OF SLEEP:

3-4 MEALS, NO SNACKING   YES/NO

2.

HUNGER 30 MINUTES BEFORE BREAKFAST   YES/NO

HUNGER 30 MIN BEFORE LUNCH   YES/NO

HUNGER 30 MIN BEFORE DINNER   YES/NO

DAILY AFFIRMATION:

AT ALL MEALS, EAT JUST ENOUGH   YES/NO

CRAVINGS AND MY REACTION TO THEM

DAILY FOOD OR BODY WIN

INTENTION SETTING FOR TOMORROW

DAILY JOURNAL

DATE

TO DO LIST:

_____

_____

_____

TODAY I AM GRATEFUL FOR:

1. _____

_____

2. _____

_____

DAILY AFFIRMATION:

_____

CRAVINGS AND MY REACTION TO THEM

_____

_____

_____

_____

INTENTION SETTING FOR TOMORROW

_____

_____

_____

WATER TRACKER   ○○○○○○○

MOVEMENT

_____

_____

MOOD TRACKER   ☹ ☹ ☺ ☺ ☺

HOURS OF SLEEP:

3-4 MEALS, NO SNACKING	YES/NO
HUNGER 30 MINUTES BEFORE BREAKFAST	YES/NO
HUNGER 30 MIN BEFORE LUNCH	YES/NO
HUNGER 30 MIN BEFORE DINNER	YES/NO
AT ALL MEALS, EAT JUST ENOUGH	YES/NO

DAILY FOOD OR BODY WIN

_____

_____

_____

_____

WEEKLY JOURNAL

DATE

WEIGHT:

MY WHY...
_____
_____
_____
_____

WHAT IS GOING WELL WITH THIS WEEKS HABIT?
_____
_____
_____
_____

WHAT COULD BE BETTER?
_____
_____
_____
_____

GOALS FOR NEXT WEEK...
_____
_____
_____
_____

DAILY JOURNAL

DATE

TO DO LIST:

_____

_____

_____

TODAY I AM GRATEFUL FOR:

1.

_____

2.

_____

DAILY AFFIRMATION:

_____

CRAVINGS AND MY REACTION TO THEM

_____

_____

_____

_____

WATER TRACKER   ⬦⬦⬦⬦⬦⬦⬦

MOVEMENT

_____

MOOD TRACKER   ☹ ☹ ☺ ☺ ☺

HOURS OF SLEEP:

3-4 MEALS, NO SNACKING	YES/NO
HUNGER 30 MINUTES BEFORE BREAKFAST	YES/NO
HUNGER 30 MIN BEFORE LUNCH	YES/NO
HUNGER 30 MIN BEFORE DINNER	YES/NO
AT ALL MEALS, EAT JUST ENOUGH	YES/NO

DAILY FOOD OR BODY WIN

_____

_____

_____

_____

INTENTION SETTING FOR TOMORROW

_____

_____

_____

DAILY JOURNAL

DATE

TO DO LIST:

_____

_____

_____

_____

TODAY I AM GRATEFUL FOR:

1. _____

_____

2. _____

_____

DAILY AFFIRMATION:

_____

CRAVINGS AND MY REACTION TO THEM

_____

_____

_____

_____

_____

INTENTION SETTING FOR TOMORROW

_____

_____

_____

WATER TRACKER ○○○○○○○

MOVEMENT

_____

_____

MOOD TRACKER ☹ ☹ ☺ ☺ ☺

HOURS OF SLEEP:

3-4 MEALS, NO SNACKING	YES/NO
HUNGER 30 MINUTES BEFORE BREAKFAST	YES/NO
HUNGER 30 MIN BEFORE LUNCH	YES/NO
HUNGER 30 MIN BEFORE DINNER	YES/NO
AT ALL MEALS, EAT JUST ENOUGH	YES/NO

DAILY FOOD OR BODY WIN

_____

_____

_____

_____

DAILY JOURNAL

DATE

TO DO LIST:

TODAY I AM GRATEFUL FOR:

1.

2.

DAILY AFFIRMATION:

CRAVINGS AND MY REACTION TO THEM

INTENTION SETTING FOR TOMORROW

WATER TRACKER ⬭⬭⬭⬭⬭⬭⬭

MOVEMENT

MOOD TRACKER ☹ 🙁 😐 🙂 😊

HOURS OF SLEEP:

3-4 MEALS, NO SNACKING	YES/NO
HUNGER 30 MINUTES BEFORE BREAKFAST	YES/NO
HUNGER 30 MIN BEFORE LUNCH	YES/NO
HUNGER 30 MIN BEFORE DINNER	YES/NO
AT ALL MEALS, EAT JUST ENOUGH	YES/NO

DAILY FOOD OR BODY WIN

DAILY JOURNAL

DATE

TO DO LIST:

_____

_____

_____

TODAY I AM GRATEFUL FOR:

1.

_____

2.

_____

DAILY AFFIRMATION:

_____

CRAVINGS AND MY REACTION TO THEM

_____

_____

_____

_____

INTENTION SETTING FOR TOMORROW

_____

_____

_____

WATER TRACKER   ◇◇◇◇◇◇◇

MOVEMENT

_____

MOOD TRACKER   ☹ ☹ ☺ ☺ ☺

HOURS OF SLEEP:

3-4 MEALS, NO SNACKING	YES/NO
HUNGER 30 MINUTES BEFORE BREAKFAST	YES/NO
HUNGER 30 MIN BEFORE LUNCH	YES/NO
HUNGER 30 MIN BEFORE DINNER	YES/NO
AT ALL MEALS, EAT JUST ENOUGH	YES/NO

DAILY FOOD OR BODY WIN

_____

_____

_____

_____

DAILY JOURNAL

DATE

_____

TO DO LIST:

_____

_____

_____

TODAY I AM GRATEFUL FOR:

1. _____

_____

2. _____

_____

DAILY AFFIRMATION:

_____

CRAVINGS AND MY REACTION TO THEM

_____

_____

_____

_____

INTENTION SETTING FOR TOMORROW

_____

_____

_____

WATER TRACKER   ◇◇◇◇◇◇◇

MOVEMENT

_____

MOOD TRACKER   ☹ ☹ 😐 ☺ ☺

HOURS OF SLEEP:

3-4 MEALS, NO SNACKING   YES/NO

HUNGER 30 MINUTES BEFORE BREAKFAST   YES/NO

HUNGER 30 MIN BEFORE LUNCH   YES/NO

HUNGER 30 MIN BEFORE DINNER   YES/NO

AT ALL MEALS, EAT JUST ENOUGH   YES/NO

DAILY FOOD OR BODY WIN

_____

_____

_____

_____

DAILY JOURNAL

DATE

TO DO LIST:

_____

_____

_____

_____

TODAY I AM GRATEFUL FOR:

1.
_____

2.
_____

DAILY AFFIRMATION:

_____

CRAVINGS AND MY REACTION TO THEM

_____

_____

_____

_____

INTENTION SETTING FOR TOMORROW

_____

_____

_____

_____

WATER TRACKER   ◊◊◊◊◊◊◊

MOVEMENT

_____

MOOD TRACKER   ☹ ☹ ☺ ☺ ☺

HOURS OF SLEEP:

3-4 MEALS, NO SNACKING	YES/NO
HUNGER 30 MINUTES BEFORE BREAKFAST	YES/NO
HUNGER 30 MIN BEFORE LUNCH	YES/NO
HUNGER 30 MIN BEFORE DINNER	YES/NO
AT ALL MEALS, EAT JUST ENOUGH	YES/NO

DAILY FOOD OR BODY WIN

_____

_____

_____

_____

DAILY JOURNAL

DATE

TO DO LIST:

_____

_____

_____

TODAY I AM GRATEFUL FOR:

1.

_____

2.

_____

DAILY AFFIRMATION:

_____

CRAVINGS AND MY REACTION TO THEM

_____

_____

_____

_____

INTENTION SETTING FOR TOMORROW

_____

_____

_____

WATER TRACKER ⬡⬡⬡⬡⬡⬡⬡

MOVEMENT

_____

MOOD TRACKER ☹ ☹ 😐 🙂 😊

HOURS OF SLEEP:

3-4 MEALS, NO SNACKING	YES/NO
HUNGER 30 MINUTES BEFORE BREAKFAST	YES/NO
HUNGER 30 MIN BEFORE LUNCH	YES/NO
HUNGER 30 MIN BEFORE DINNER	YES/NO
AT ALL MEALS, EAT JUST ENOUGH	YES/NO

DAILY FOOD OR BODY WIN

_____

_____

_____

_____

WEEKLY JOURNAL

DATE

WEIGHT:

MY WHY...
_____
_____
_____
_____

WHAT IS GOING WELL WITH THIS WEEKS HABIT?
_____
_____
_____

WHAT COULD BE BETTER?
_____
_____
_____

GOALS FOR NEXT WEEK...
_____
_____
_____

DAILY JOURNAL

DATE

TO DO LIST:

WATER TRACKER ⬭⬭⬭⬭⬭⬭⬭

MOVEMENT

TODAY I AM GRATEFUL FOR:

MOOD TRACKER ☹ ☹ ☺ ☺ ☺

HOURS OF SLEEP:

1.

3-4 MEALS, NO SNACKING	YES/NO

HUNGER 30 MINUTES BEFORE BREAKFAST	YES/NO

2.

HUNGER 30 MIN BEFORE LUNCH	YES/NO

HUNGER 30 MIN BEFORE DINNER	YES/NO

DAILY AFFIRMATION:

AT ALL MEALS, EAT JUST ENOUGH	YES/NO

CRAVINGS AND MY REACTION TO THEM

DAILY FOOD OR BODY WIN

INTENTION SETTING FOR TOMORROW

DAILY JOURNAL

DATE

TO DO LIST:

WATER TRACKER   ○○○○○○○

MOVEMENT

MOOD TRACKER   ☹ ☹ ☺ ☺ ☺

TODAY I AM GRATEFUL FOR:

HOURS OF SLEEP:

1.

3-4 MEALS, NO SNACKING   YES/NO

2.

HUNGER 30 MIN BEFORE LUNCH   YES/NO

HUNGER 30 MIN BEFORE DINNER   YES/NO

DAILY AFFIRMATION:

AT ALL MEALS, EAT JUST ENOUGH   YES/NO

CRAVINGS AND MY REACTION TO THEM

DAILY FOOD OR BODY WIN

INTENTION SETTING FOR TOMORROW

DAILY JOURNAL

DATE

TO DO LIST:

_____

_____

_____

TODAY I AM GRATEFUL FOR:

1. _____

2. _____

DAILY AFFIRMATION:

_____

CRAVINGS AND MY REACTION TO THEM

_____

_____

_____

_____

INTENTION SETTING FOR TOMORROW

_____

_____

_____

WATER TRACKER ⬡⬡⬡⬡⬡⬡⬡

MOVEMENT

_____

MOOD TRACKER ☹ ☹ ☺ ☺ ☺

HOURS OF SLEEP:

3-4 MEALS, NO SNACKING	YES/NO
HUNGER 30 MINUTES BEFORE BREAKFAST	YES/NO
HUNGER 30 MIN BEFORE LUNCH	YES/NO
HUNGER 30 MIN BEFORE DINNER	YES/NO
AT ALL MEALS, EAT JUST ENOUGH	YES/NO

DAILY FOOD OR BODY WIN

_____

_____

_____

_____

DAILY JOURNAL

DATE

TO DO LIST:

_____

_____

_____

_____

TODAY I AM GRATEFUL FOR:

1. _____

_____

2. _____

_____

DAILY AFFIRMATION:

_____

CRAVINGS AND MY REACTION TO THEM

_____

_____

_____

_____

WATER TRACKER   ⬡⬡⬡⬡⬡⬡⬡

MOVEMENT

_____

MOOD TRACKER   ☹ ☹ ☺ ☺ ☺

HOURS OF SLEEP:

3-4 MEALS, NO SNACKING	YES/NO
HUNGER 30 MINUTES BEFORE BREAKFAST	YES/NO
HUNGER 30 MIN BEFORE LUNCH	YES/NO
HUNGER 30 MIN BEFORE DINNER	YES/NO
AT ALL MEALS, EAT JUST ENOUGH	YES/NO

DAILY FOOD OR BODY WIN

_____

_____

_____

_____

INTENTION SETTING FOR TOMORROW

_____

_____

_____

DAILY JOURNAL

DATE

TO DO LIST:

_____

_____

_____

TODAY I AM GRATEFUL FOR:

1. _____

_____

2. _____

_____

DAILY AFFIRMATION:

_____

CRAVINGS AND MY REACTION TO THEM

_____

_____

_____

_____

_____

INTENTION SETTING FOR TOMORROW

_____

_____

_____

_____

WATER TRACKER   ◌◌◌◌◌◌◌

MOVEMENT

_____

MOOD TRACKER   ☹ ☹ ☺ ☺ ☺

HOURS OF SLEEP:

3-4 MEALS, NO SNACKING   YES/NO

HUNGER 30 MINUTES BEFORE BREAKFAST   YES/NO

HUNGER 30 MIN BEFORE LUNCH   YES/NO

HUNGER 30 MIN BEFORE DINNER   YES/NO

AT ALL MEALS, EAT JUST ENOUGH   YES/NO

DAILY FOOD OR BODY WIN

_____

_____

_____

_____

_____

DAILY JOURNAL

DATE

TO DO LIST:

_____

_____

_____

_____

TODAY I AM GRATEFUL FOR:

1. _____

_____

2. _____

_____

DAILY AFFIRMATION:

_____

CRAVINGS AND MY REACTION TO THEM

_____

_____

_____

_____

WATER TRACKER ◇◇◇◇◇◇◇

MOVEMENT

_____

_____

MOOD TRACKER ☹ ☹ ☺ ☺ ☺

HOURS OF SLEEP:

3-4 MEALS, NO SNACKING	YES/NO
HUNGER 30 MINUTES BEFORE BREAKFAST	YES/NO
HUNGER 30 MIN BEFORE LUNCH	YES/NO
HUNGER 30 MIN BEFORE DINNER	YES/NO
AT ALL MEALS, EAT JUST ENOUGH	YES/NO

DAILY FOOD OR BODY WIN

_____

_____

_____

_____

INTENTION SETTING FOR TOMORROW

_____

_____

_____

DAILY JOURNAL

DATE

TO DO LIST:

_____

_____

_____

_____

TODAY I AM GRATEFUL FOR:

1. _____

_____

2. _____

_____

DAILY AFFIRMATION:

_____

CRAVINGS AND MY REACTION TO THEM

_____

_____

_____

_____

WATER TRACKER ○○○○○○○

MOVEMENT

_____

_____

MOOD TRACKER ☹ ☹ ☺ ☺ ☺

HOURS OF SLEEP:

3-4 MEALS, NO SNACKING   YES/NO

HUNGER 30 MINUTES BEFORE BREAKFAST   YES/NO

HUNGER 30 MIN BEFORE LUNCH   YES/NO

HUNGER 30 MIN BEFORE DINNER   YES/NO

AT ALL MEALS, EAT JUST ENOUGH   YES/NO

DAILY FOOD OR BODY WIN

_____

_____

_____

_____

INTENTION SETTING FOR TOMORROW

_____

_____

_____

_____

WEEKLY JOURNAL

DATE

WEIGHT:

MY WHY...

_____
_____
_____
_____

WHAT IS GOING WELL WITH THIS WEEKS HABIT?

_____
_____
_____
_____

WHAT COULD BE BETTER?

_____
_____
_____
_____

GOALS FOR NEXT WEEK...

_____
_____
_____
_____

MONTHLY JOURNAL

DATE

_____

MEASUREMENTS-
_____

CHEST:
_____

WAIST:
_____

HIPS:
_____

THIGHS: RIGHT-   LEFT-
_____

CALF: RIGHT-   LEFT-
_____

ARMS: RIGHT-   LEFT-
_____

LOOK HOW FAR I'VE COME!!
WRITE DOWN EXAMPLES OF WAYS YOU HAVE IMPROVED IN THE LAST 4 WEEKS

_____

_____

_____

_____

_____

_____

_____

_____

_____

_____

DAILY JOURNAL

DATE

TO DO LIST:

_____

_____

_____

TODAY I AM GRATEFUL FOR:

1.

_____

2.

_____

DAILY AFFIRMATION:

_____

CRAVINGS AND MY REACTION TO THEM

_____

_____

_____

_____

_____

INTENTION SETTING FOR TOMORROW

_____

_____

_____

WATER TRACKER   ○○○○○○○

MOVEMENT

_____

MOOD TRACKER   ☹ ☹ ☺ ☺ ☺

HOURS OF SLEEP:

3-4 MEALS, NO SNACKING	YES/NO
HUNGER 30 MINUTES BEFORE BREAKFAST	YES/NO
HUNGER 30 MIN BEFORE LUNCH	YES/NO
HUNGER 30 MIN BEFORE DINNER	YES/NO
AT ALL MEALS, EAT JUST ENOUGH	YES/NO

DAILY FOOD OR BODY WIN

_____

_____

_____

_____

_____

DAILY JOURNAL

DATE

TO DO LIST:

WATER TRACKER ⬡⬡⬡⬡⬡⬡⬡

MOVEMENT

TODAY I AM GRATEFUL FOR:

MOOD TRACKER ☹ ☹ ☺ ☺ ☺

HOURS OF SLEEP:

1.

3-4 MEALS, NO SNACKING	YES/NO
HUNGER 30 MINUTES BEFORE BREAKFAST	YES/NO
HUNGER 30 MIN BEFORE LUNCH	YES/NO

2.

HUNGER 30 MIN BEFORE DINNER	YES/NO
AT ALL MEALS, EAT JUST ENOUGH	YES/NO

DAILY AFFIRMATION:

CRAVINGS AND MY REACTION TO THEM

DAILY FOOD OR BODY WIN

INTENTION SETTING FOR TOMORROW

DAILY JOURNAL

DATE

TO DO LIST:

_____

_____

_____

WATER TRACKER　　　△△△△△△△

MOVEMENT

_____

MOOD TRACKER　　　☹ ☹ 😐 ☺ ☺

HOURS OF SLEEP:

TODAY I AM GRATEFUL FOR:

1.

_____

2.

_____

3-4 MEALS, NO SNACKING	YES/NO
HUNGER 30 MINUTES BEFORE BREAKFAST	YES/NO
HUNGER 30 MIN BEFORE LUNCH	YES/NO
HUNGER 30 MIN BEFORE DINNER	YES/NO
AT ALL MEALS, EAT JUST ENOUGH	YES/NO

DAILY AFFIRMATION:

_____

CRAVINGS AND MY REACTION TO THEM

_____

_____

_____

_____

DAILY FOOD OR BODY WIN

_____

_____

_____

_____

INTENTION SETTING FOR TOMORROW

_____

_____

_____

DAILY JOURNAL

DATE

TO DO LIST:

_____

_____

_____

_____

TODAY I AM GRATEFUL FOR:

1. _____

_____

2. _____

_____

DAILY AFFIRMATION:

_____

CRAVINGS AND MY REACTION TO THEM

_____

_____

_____

_____

INTENTION SETTING FOR TOMORROW

_____

_____

_____

WATER TRACKER ◇◇◇◇◇◇◇

MOVEMENT

_____

_____

MOOD TRACKER ☹ ☹ ☺ ☺ ☺

HOURS OF SLEEP:

3-4 MEALS, NO SNACKING	YES/NO
HUNGER 30 MINUTES BEFORE BREAKFAST	YES/NO
HUNGER 30 MIN BEFORE LUNCH	YES/NO
HUNGER 30 MIN BEFORE DINNER	YES/NO
AT ALL MEALS, EAT JUST ENOUGH	YES/NO

DAILY FOOD OR BODY WIN

_____

_____

_____

_____

DAILY JOURNAL

DATE

TO DO LIST:

WATER TRACKER   ○○○○○○○

MOVEMENT

MOOD TRACKER   ☹ ☹ 😐 🙂 😊

TODAY I AM GRATEFUL FOR:

HOURS OF SLEEP:

1.

3-4 MEALS, NO SNACKING	YES/NO
HUNGER 30 MINUTES BEFORE BREAKFAST	YES/NO
HUNGER 30 MIN BEFORE LUNCH	YES/NO
HUNGER 30 MIN BEFORE DINNER	YES/NO
AT ALL MEALS, EAT JUST ENOUGH	YES/NO

2.

DAILY AFFIRMATION:

CRAVINGS AND MY REACTION TO THEM

DAILY FOOD OR BODY WIN

INTENTION SETTING FOR TOMORROW

DAILY JOURNAL

DATE

TO DO LIST:

_____

_____

_____

TODAY I AM GRATEFUL FOR:

1.

_____

2.

_____

DAILY AFFIRMATION:

_____

CRAVINGS AND MY REACTION TO THEM

_____

_____

_____

_____

INTENTION SETTING FOR TOMORROW

_____

_____

_____

WATER TRACKER ⬡⬡⬡⬡⬡⬡⬡

MOVEMENT

_____

MOOD TRACKER ☹ ☹ ☺ ☺ ☺

HOURS OF SLEEP:

3-4 MEALS, NO SNACKING	YES/NO
HUNGER 30 MINUTES BEFORE BREAKFAST	YES/NO
HUNGER 30 MIN BEFORE LUNCH	YES/NO
HUNGER 30 MIN BEFORE DINNER	YES/NO
AT ALL MEALS, EAT JUST ENOUGH	YES/NO

DAILY FOOD OR BODY WIN

_____

_____

_____

_____

DAILY JOURNAL

DATE

TO DO LIST:

_____

_____

_____

TODAY I AM GRATEFUL FOR:

1. _____

2. _____

DAILY AFFIRMATION:

_____

CRAVINGS AND MY REACTION TO THEM

_____

_____

_____

_____

INTENTION SETTING FOR TOMORROW

_____

_____

_____

WATER TRACKER ⬯⬯⬯⬯⬯⬯⬯

MOVEMENT

_____

MOOD TRACKER ☹ ☹ 😐 ☺ ☺

HOURS OF SLEEP:

3-4 MEALS, NO SNACKING	YES/NO
HUNGER 30 MINUTES BEFORE BREAKFAST	YES/NO
HUNGER 30 MIN BEFORE LUNCH	YES/NO
HUNGER 30 MIN BEFORE DINNER	YES/NO
AT ALL MEALS, EAT JUST ENOUGH	YES/NO

DAILY FOOD OR BODY WIN

_____

_____

_____

_____

WEEKLY JOURNAL

WEIGHT:

MY WHY...

_____

_____

_____

_____

WHAT IS GOING WELL WITH THIS WEEKS HABIT?

_____

_____

_____

_____

WHAT COULD BE BETTER?

_____

_____

_____

_____

GOALS FOR NEXT WEEK...

_____

_____

_____

_____

DAILY JOURNAL

DATE

TO DO LIST:

_____

_____

_____

TODAY I AM GRATEFUL FOR:

1. _____

_____

2. _____

_____

DAILY AFFIRMATION:

_____

CRAVINGS AND MY REACTION TO THEM

_____

_____

_____

_____

WATER TRACKER   ◇◇◇◇◇◇◇

MOVEMENT

_____

MOOD TRACKER   ☹ ☹ ☺ ☺ ☺

HOURS OF SLEEP:

3-4 MEALS, NO SNACKING	YES/NO
HUNGER 30 MINUTES BEFORE BREAKFAST	YES/NO
HUNGER 30 MIN BEFORE LUNCH	YES/NO
HUNGER 30 MIN BEFORE DINNER	YES/NO
AT ALL MEALS, EAT JUST ENOUGH	YES/NO

DAILY FOOD OR BODY WIN

_____

_____

_____

_____

INTENTION SETTING FOR TOMORROW

_____

_____

_____

DAILY JOURNAL

DATE

TO DO LIST:

WATER TRACKER ⬠⬠⬠⬠⬠⬠⬠

MOVEMENT

MOOD TRACKER ☹ ☹ ☺ ☺ ☺

TODAY I AM GRATEFUL FOR:

HOURS OF SLEEP:

1.

3-4 MEALS, NO SNACKING	YES/NO
HUNGER 30 MINUTES BEFORE BREAKFAST	YES/NO
HUNGER 30 MIN BEFORE LUNCH	YES/NO
HUNGER 30 MIN BEFORE DINNER	YES/NO
AT ALL MEALS, EAT JUST ENOUGH	YES/NO

2.

DAILY AFFIRMATION:

CRAVINGS AND MY REACTION TO THEM

DAILY FOOD OR BODY WIN

INTENTION SETTING FOR TOMORROW

DAILY JOURNAL

DATE

TO DO LIST:

_____

_____

_____

_____

TODAY I AM GRATEFUL FOR:

1. _____

_____

2. _____

_____

DAILY AFFIRMATION:

_____

CRAVINGS AND MY REACTION TO THEM

_____

_____

_____

_____

_____

WATER TRACKER ○○○○○○○

MOVEMENT

_____

_____

MOOD TRACKER ☹ ☹ 😐 ☺ 😊

HOURS OF SLEEP:

3-4 MEALS, NO SNACKING	YES/NO
HUNGER 30 MINUTES BEFORE BREAKFAST	YES/NO
HUNGER 30 MIN BEFORE LUNCH	YES/NO
HUNGER 30 MIN BEFORE DINNER	YES/NO
AT ALL MEALS, EAT JUST ENOUGH	YES/NO

DAILY FOOD OR BODY WIN

_____

_____

_____

_____

INTENTION SETTING FOR TOMORROW

_____

_____

_____

_____

DAILY JOURNAL

DATE

TO DO LIST:

_____

_____

_____

TODAY I AM GRATEFUL FOR:

1. _____

_____

2. _____

_____

DAILY AFFIRMATION:

_____

CRAVINGS AND MY REACTION TO THEM

_____

_____

_____

_____

WATER TRACKER ⬡⬡⬡⬡⬡⬡⬡

MOVEMENT

_____

MOOD TRACKER ☹ 🙁 😐 🙂 😊

HOURS OF SLEEP:

3-4 MEALS, NO SNACKING	YES/NO
HUNGER 30 MINUTES BEFORE BREAKFAST	YES/NO
HUNGER 30 MIN BEFORE LUNCH	YES/NO
HUNGER 30 MIN BEFORE DINNER	YES/NO
AT ALL MEALS, EAT JUST ENOUGH	YES/NO

DAILY FOOD OR BODY WIN

_____

_____

_____

_____

INTENTION SETTING FOR TOMORROW

_____

_____

_____

DAILY JOURNAL

DATE

TO DO LIST:

WATER TRACKER ◇◇◇◇◇◇◇

MOVEMENT

TODAY I AM GRATEFUL FOR:

MOOD TRACKER ☹ ☹ ☺ ☺ ☺

HOURS OF SLEEP:

1.

| 3-4 MEALS, NO SNACKING | YES/NO |

2.

| HUNGER 30 MINUTES BEFORE BREAKFAST | YES/NO |

| HUNGER 30 MIN BEFORE LUNCH | YES/NO |

| HUNGER 30 MIN BEFORE DINNER | YES/NO |

DAILY AFFIRMATION:

| AT ALL MEALS, EAT JUST ENOUGH | YES/NO |

CRAVINGS AND MY REACTION TO THEM

DAILY FOOD OR BODY WIN

INTENTION SETTING FOR TOMORROW

DAILY JOURNAL

DATE

TO DO LIST:

_____

_____

_____

TODAY I AM GRATEFUL FOR:

1. _____

_____

2. _____

_____

DAILY AFFIRMATION:

_____

CRAVINGS AND MY REACTION TO THEM

_____

_____

_____

_____

WATER TRACKER ⬡⬡⬡⬡⬡⬡⬡

MOVEMENT

_____

_____

MOOD TRACKER ☹ ☹ ☺ ☺ ☺

HOURS OF SLEEP:

3-4 MEALS, NO SNACKING	YES/NO
HUNGER 30 MINUTES BEFORE BREAKFAST	YES/NO
HUNGER 30 MIN BEFORE LUNCH	YES/NO
HUNGER 30 MIN BEFORE DINNER	YES/NO
AT ALL MEALS, EAT JUST ENOUGH	YES/NO

DAILY FOOD OR BODY WIN

_____

_____

_____

_____

INTENTION SETTING FOR TOMORROW

_____

_____

_____

DAILY JOURNAL

DATE

TO DO LIST:

_____

_____

_____

TODAY I AM GRATEFUL FOR:

1.
_____

2.
_____

DAILY AFFIRMATION:

_____

CRAVINGS AND MY REACTION TO THEM

_____

_____

_____

_____

WATER TRACKER ◊◊◊◊◊◊◊

MOVEMENT

_____

MOOD TRACKER ☹ ☹ ☺ ☺ ☺

HOURS OF SLEEP:

3-4 MEALS, NO SNACKING	YES/NO
HUNGER 30 MINUTES BEFORE BREAKFAST	YES/NO
HUNGER 30 MIN BEFORE LUNCH	YES/NO
HUNGER 30 MIN BEFORE DINNER	YES/NO
AT ALL MEALS, EAT JUST ENOUGH	YES/NO

DAILY FOOD OR BODY WIN

_____

_____

_____

_____

INTENTION SETTING FOR TOMORROW

_____

_____

_____

WEEKLY JOURNAL

DATE

WEIGHT:

MY WHY...
_____
_____
_____
_____

WHAT IS GOING WELL WITH THIS WEEKS HABIT?
_____
_____
_____
_____

WHAT COULD BE BETTER?
_____
_____
_____
_____

GOALS FOR NEXT WEEK...
_____
_____
_____
_____

DAILY JOURNAL

DATE

TO DO LIST:

_____

_____

_____

TODAY I AM GRATEFUL FOR:

1. _____

_____

2. _____

_____

DAILY AFFIRMATION:

_____

CRAVINGS AND MY REACTION TO THEM

_____

_____

_____

_____

WATER TRACKER ○○○○○○○

MOVEMENT

_____

MOOD TRACKER ☹ ☹ ☺ ☺ ☺

HOURS OF SLEEP:

3-4 MEALS, NO SNACKING	YES/NO
HUNGER 30 MINUTES BEFORE BREAKFAST	YES/NO
HUNGER 30 MIN BEFORE LUNCH	YES/NO
HUNGER 30 MIN BEFORE DINNER	YES/NO
AT ALL MEALS, EAT JUST ENOUGH	YES/NO

DAILY FOOD OR BODY WIN

_____

_____

_____

_____

INTENTION SETTING FOR TOMORROW

_____

_____

_____

DAILY JOURNAL

DATE

TO DO LIST:

_____

_____

_____

TODAY I AM GRATEFUL FOR:

1. _____

_____

2. _____

_____

DAILY AFFIRMATION:

_____

CRAVINGS AND MY REACTION TO THEM

_____

_____

_____

_____

WATER TRACKER ⬡⬡⬡⬡⬡⬡⬡

MOVEMENT

_____

_____

MOOD TRACKER ☹ ☹ ☺ ☺ ☺

HOURS OF SLEEP:

3-4 MEALS, NO SNACKING	YES/NO
HUNGER 30 MINUTES BEFORE BREAKFAST	YES/NO
HUNGER 30 MIN BEFORE LUNCH	YES/NO
HUNGER 30 MIN BEFORE DINNER	YES/NO
AT ALL MEALS, EAT JUST ENOUGH	YES/NO

DAILY FOOD OR BODY WIN

_____

_____

_____

INTENTION SETTING FOR TOMORROW

_____

_____

_____

DAILY JOURNAL

DATE

TO DO LIST:

_____

_____

_____

_____

TODAY I AM GRATEFUL FOR:

1.

_____

2.

_____

DAILY AFFIRMATION:

_____

CRAVINGS AND MY REACTION TO THEM

_____

_____

_____

_____

WATER TRACKER ○○○○○○○

MOVEMENT

_____

_____

MOOD TRACKER ☹ ☹ ☺ ☺ ☺

HOURS OF SLEEP:

3-4 MEALS, NO SNACKING	YES/NO
HUNGER 30 MINUTES BEFORE BREAKFAST	YES/NO
HUNGER 30 MIN BEFORE LUNCH	YES/NO
HUNGER 30 MIN BEFORE DINNER	YES/NO
AT ALL MEALS, EAT JUST ENOUGH	YES/NO

DAILY FOOD OR BODY WIN

_____

_____

_____

_____

INTENTION SETTING FOR TOMORROW

_____

_____

_____

DAILY JOURNAL

DATE

TO DO LIST:

WATER TRACKER   ○○○○○○○

MOVEMENT

TODAY I AM GRATEFUL FOR:

MOOD TRACKER   ☹ ☹ ☺ ☺ ☺

HOURS OF SLEEP:

1.

3-4 MEALS, NO SNACKING	YES/NO
HUNGER 30 MINUTES BEFORE BREAKFAST	YES/NO
HUNGER 30 MIN BEFORE LUNCH	YES/NO
HUNGER 30 MIN BEFORE DINNER	YES/NO
AT ALL MEALS, EAT JUST ENOUGH	YES/NO

2.

DAILY AFFIRMATION:

CRAVINGS AND MY REACTION TO THEM

DAILY FOOD OR BODY WIN

INTENTION SETTING FOR TOMORROW

DAILY JOURNAL

DATE

TO DO LIST:

_____

_____

_____

TODAY I AM GRATEFUL FOR:

1.

_____

2.

_____

DAILY AFFIRMATION:

_____

CRAVINGS AND MY REACTION TO THEM

_____

_____

_____

_____

WATER TRACKER ◌◌◌◌◌◌◌

MOVEMENT

_____

MOOD TRACKER ☹ ☹ ☺ ☺ ☺

HOURS OF SLEEP:

3-4 MEALS, NO SNACKING	YES/NO
HUNGER 30 MINUTES BEFORE BREAKFAST	YES/NO
HUNGER 30 MIN BEFORE LUNCH	YES/NO
HUNGER 30 MIN BEFORE DINNER	YES/NO
AT ALL MEALS, EAT JUST ENOUGH	YES/NO

DAILY FOOD OR BODY WIN

_____

_____

_____

_____

INTENTION SETTING FOR TOMORROW

_____

_____

_____

DAILY JOURNAL

DATE

TO DO LIST:

WATER TRACKER ⬭⬭⬭⬭⬭⬭⬭

MOVEMENT

TODAY I AM GRATEFUL FOR:

MOOD TRACKER ☹ ☹ 😐 ☺ ☺

HOURS OF SLEEP:

1.

3-4 MEALS, NO SNACKING   YES/NO

HUNGER 30 MINUTES BEFORE BREAKFAST   YES/NO

2.

HUNGER 30 MIN BEFORE LUNCH   YES/NO

HUNGER 30 MIN BEFORE DINNER   YES/NO

DAILY AFFIRMATION:

AT ALL MEALS, EAT JUST ENOUGH   YES/NO

CRAVINGS AND MY REACTION TO THEM

DAILY FOOD OR BODY WIN

INTENTION SETTING FOR TOMORROW

DAILY JOURNAL

DATE

TO DO LIST:

_____

_____

_____

TODAY I AM GRATEFUL FOR:

1.

_____

2.

_____

DAILY AFFIRMATION:

_____

CRAVINGS AND MY REACTION TO THEM

_____

_____

_____

_____

INTENTION SETTING FOR TOMORROW

_____

_____

_____

WATER TRACKER ◊◊◊◊◊◊◊

MOVEMENT

_____

MOOD TRACKER ☹ ☹ ☺ ☺ ☺

HOURS OF SLEEP:

3-4 MEALS, NO SNACKING	YES/NO
HUNGER 30 MINUTES BEFORE BREAKFAST	YES/NO
HUNGER 30 MIN BEFORE LUNCH	YES/NO
HUNGER 30 MIN BEFORE DINNER	YES/NO
AT ALL MEALS, EAT JUST ENOUGH	YES/NO

DAILY FOOD OR BODY WIN

_____

_____

_____

_____

WEEKLY JOURNAL

DATE

WEIGHT:

MY WHY...
_____
_____
_____
_____

WHAT IS GOING WELL WITH THIS WEEKS HABIT?
_____
_____
_____
_____

WHAT COULD BE BETTER?
_____
_____
_____
_____

GOALS FOR NEXT WEEK...
_____
_____
_____
_____

DAILY JOURNAL

DATE

TO DO LIST:

_____

_____

_____

_____

WATER TRACKER ◇◇◇◇◇◇◇

MOVEMENT

_____

_____

TODAY I AM GRATEFUL FOR:

1.

_____

_____

2.

_____

_____

DAILY AFFIRMATION:

_____

_____

MOOD TRACKER ☹ ☹ ☺ ☺ ☺

HOURS OF SLEEP:

3-4 MEALS, NO SNACKING	YES/NO
HUNGER 30 MINUTES BEFORE BREAKFAST	YES/NO
HUNGER 30 MIN BEFORE LUNCH	YES/NO
HUNGER 30 MIN BEFORE DINNER	YES/NO
AT ALL MEALS, EAT JUST ENOUGH	YES/NO

CRAVINGS AND MY REACTION TO THEM

_____

_____

_____

_____

_____

DAILY FOOD OR BODY WIN

_____

_____

_____

_____

_____

INTENTION SETTING FOR TOMORROW

_____

_____

_____

_____

DAILY JOURNAL

DATE

TO DO LIST:

WATER TRACKER ○○○○○○○

MOVEMENT

TODAY I AM GRATEFUL FOR:

MOOD TRACKER ☹ ☹ ☺ ☺ ☺

HOURS OF SLEEP:

1.

| 3-4 MEALS, NO SNACKING | YES/NO |
| HUNGER 30 MINUTES BEFORE BREAKFAST | YES/NO |

2.

| HUNGER 30 MIN BEFORE LUNCH | YES/NO |
| HUNGER 30 MIN BEFORE DINNER | YES/NO |

DAILY AFFIRMATION:

AT ALL MEALS, EAT JUST ENOUGH   YES/NO

CRAVINGS AND MY REACTION TO THEM

DAILY FOOD OR BODY WIN

INTENTION SETTING FOR TOMORROW

DAILY JOURNAL

DATE

TO DO LIST:

WATER TRACKER ⬦⬦⬦⬦⬦⬦⬦

MOVEMENT

MOOD TRACKER ☹ ☹ ☺ ☺ ☺

TODAY I AM GRATEFUL FOR:

HOURS OF SLEEP:

1.

3-4 MEALS, NO SNACKING   YES/NO

HUNGER 30 MINUTES BEFORE BREAKFAST   YES/NO

2.

HUNGER 30 MIN BEFORE LUNCH   YES/NO

HUNGER 30 MIN BEFORE DINNER   YES/NO

DAILY AFFIRMATION:

AT ALL MEALS, EAT JUST ENOUGH   YES/NO

CRAVINGS AND MY REACTION TO THEM

DAILY FOOD OR BODY WIN

INTENTION SETTING FOR TOMORROW

DAILY JOURNAL

DATE

TO DO LIST:

WATER TRACKER   ◊◊◊◊◊◊◊

MOVEMENT

MOOD TRACKER   ☹ ☹ ☺ ☺ ☺

TODAY I AM GRATEFUL FOR:

HOURS OF SLEEP:

1.

3-4 MEALS, NO SNACKING   YES/NO

HUNGER 30 MINUTES BEFORE BREAKFAST   YES/NO

2.

HUNGER 30 MIN BEFORE LUNCH   YES/NO

HUNGER 30 MIN BEFORE DINNER   YES/NO

DAILY AFFIRMATION:

AT ALL MEALS, EAT JUST ENOUGH   YES/NO

CRAVINGS AND MY REACTION TO THEM

DAILY FOOD OR BODY WIN

INTENTION SETTING FOR TOMORROW

DAILY JOURNAL

DATE

TO DO LIST:

_____

_____

_____

_____

TODAY I AM GRATEFUL FOR:

1. _____

_____

2. _____

_____

DAILY AFFIRMATION:

_____

CRAVINGS AND MY REACTION TO THEM

_____

_____

_____

_____

INTENTION SETTING FOR TOMORROW

_____

_____

_____

_____

WATER TRACKER ⬡⬡⬡⬡⬡⬡⬡

MOVEMENT

_____

_____

MOOD TRACKER ☹ ☹ 😐 ☺ ☺

HOURS OF SLEEP:

3-4 MEALS, NO SNACKING   YES/NO

HUNGER 30 MINUTES BEFORE BREAKFAST   YES/NO

HUNGER 30 MIN BEFORE LUNCH   YES/NO

HUNGER 30 MIN BEFORE DINNER   YES/NO

AT ALL MEALS, EAT JUST ENOUGH   YES/NO

DAILY FOOD OR BODY WIN

_____

_____

_____

_____

DAILY JOURNAL

DATE

TO DO LIST:

_____

_____

_____

_____

TODAY I AM GRATEFUL FOR:

1. _____

_____

2. _____

_____

DAILY AFFIRMATION:

_____

CRAVINGS AND MY REACTION TO THEM

_____

_____

_____

_____

INTENTION SETTING FOR TOMORROW

_____

_____

_____

WATER TRACKER ○○○○○○○

MOVEMENT

_____

_____

MOOD TRACKER ☹ ☹ ☺ ☺ ☺

HOURS OF SLEEP:

3-4 MEALS, NO SNACKING	YES/NO
HUNGER 30 MINUTES BEFORE BREAKFAST	YES/NO
HUNGER 30 MIN BEFORE LUNCH	YES/NO
HUNGER 30 MIN BEFORE DINNER	YES/NO
AT ALL MEALS, EAT JUST ENOUGH	YES/NO

DAILY FOOD OR BODY WIN

_____

_____

_____

_____

DAILY JOURNAL

DATE

TO DO LIST:

_____

_____

_____

TODAY I AM GRATEFUL FOR:

1.

_____

2.

_____

DAILY AFFIRMATION:

_____

CRAVINGS AND MY REACTION TO THEM

_____

_____

_____

_____

INTENTION SETTING FOR TOMORROW

_____

_____

_____

WATER TRACKER ◊◊◊◊◊◊◊

MOVEMENT

_____

MOOD TRACKER ☹ ☹ ☺ ☺ ☺

HOURS OF SLEEP:

3-4 MEALS, NO SNACKING	YES/NO
HUNGER 30 MINUTES BEFORE BREAKFAST	YES/NO
HUNGER 30 MIN BEFORE LUNCH	YES/NO
HUNGER 30 MIN BEFORE DINNER	YES/NO
AT ALL MEALS, EAT JUST ENOUGH	YES/NO

DAILY FOOD OR BODY WIN

_____

_____

_____

_____

WEEKLY JOURNAL

DATE

WEIGHT:

MY WHY...
_____

_____

_____

_____

WHAT IS GOING WELL WITH THIS WEEKS HABIT?
_____

_____

_____

_____

WHAT COULD BE BETTER?
_____

_____

_____

_____

GOALS FOR NEXT WEEK...
_____

_____

_____

_____

MONTHLY JOURNAL

DATE

MEASUREMENTS-

CHEST:

WAIST:

HIPS:

THIGHS: RIGHT-   LEFT-

CALF: RIGHT-   LEFT-

ARMS: RIGHT-   LEFT-

LOOK HOW FAR I'VE COME!!
WRITE DOWN EXAMPLES OF WAYS YOU HAVE IMPROVED IN THE LAST 4 WEEKS

RESOURCES

EDDINS, R. (2022, MAY 4). BUILD A POSITIVE BODY IMAGE THROUGH BODY ACCEPTANCE EXERCISES & SELF TALK. EDDINS COUNSELING GROUP – HOUSTON & SUGAR LAND, TX. HTTPS://EDDINSCOUNSELING.COM/BODY-ACCEPTANCE-EXERCISE/

FEAR, G. (2015). LEAN HABITS FOR LIFELONG WEIGHT LOSS: MASTERING 4 CORE EATING BEHAVIORS TO STAY SLIM FOREVER. PAGE STREET PUBLISHING.

FEAR, G. (2020). GIVE YOURSELF MORE: A SCIENCE-BACKED, SIX-PART PLAN FOR WOMEN TO HIT THEIR WEIGH.

PATUREL, A. (2014, JULY 6). SLEEP MORE, WEIGH LESS. WEBMD. HTTPS://WWW.WEBMD.COM/DIET/SLEEP-AND-WEIGHT-LOSS

RAVIKANT, K. (2020). LOVE YOURSELF LIKE YOUR LIFE DEPENDS ON IT. HARPERCOLLINS.

TEPEDINO, K. (2014, DECEMBER 27). CHANGE THIS ONE THOUGHT AND LOSE WEIGHT. HUFFPOST. HTTPS://WWW.HUFFPOST.COM/ENTRY/CHANGE-THIS-ONE-THOUGHT-L_B_6043274

WILE. (N.D.). UNDERSTANDING EMOTIONAL EATING & STEPS TO OVERCOME IT. HTTPS://WILEWOMEN.COM/BLOGS/JOURNAL/EMOTIONAL-EATING-DURING-STRESSFUL-TIMES-AND-THE-STEPS-TO-OVERCOME-IT? GAD=1&GCLID=CJ0KCQJWR82IBHCUARISAO0EAZYUMLRX8EBBS-PUVNSORS7TGKP4QKGLUEI-5MA5S7CKEV2XTJGUYCSAAS7PEALW_WCB

YES, DRINKING MORE WATER MAY HELP YOU LOSE WEIGHT. (2020, JANUARY 15). THE HUB. HTTPS://HUB.JHU.EDU/AT-WORK/2020/01/15/FOCUS-ON-WELLNESS-DRINKING-MORE-WATER/

Printed in the USA
CPSIA information can be obtained
at www.ICGtesting.com
LVHW011122131023
760817LV00020B/1519

9 798988 812906